12/90

Best wishes for a joyous holiday season and a happy New Year!

ESSENTIALS OF GERIATRIC PSYCHIATRY: A GUIDE FOR HEALTH PROFESSIONALS

AMERICAN ASSOCIATION FOR GERIATRIC PSYCHIATRY
Editorial Committee

Lawrence W. Lazarus, M.D., *Editor*
Assistant Professor of Psychiatry
Rush Medical College
Chicago, Illinois

Lissy F. Jarvik, M.D., Ph.D., *Consulting Editor*
Professor, Department of Psychiatry and Behavioral Sciences and
Chief, Section on Neuro-psychogeriatrics
Neuropsychiatric Institute and Hospital
University of California, Los Angeles and
Chief, Psychogeriatric Unit
West Los Angeles Veterans Administration Medical Center, Brentwood Division
Los Angeles, California

Jeffrey R. Foster, M.D.
Director of Geriatric Services and Training Program
Department of Psychiatry
New York University Medical Center
New York, New York

Jonathan D. Lieff, M.D.
Associate Clinical Professor of Psychiatry
Boston University Medical School and
Chief of Psychiatry, Hahnemann Hospital
Boston, Massachusetts

Steven R. Mershon, M.D.
Assistant Professor of Psychiatry
Rush Medical College
Chicago, Illinois

Essentials of Geriatric Psychiatry
A Guide for Health Professionals

Lawrence W. Lazarus, M.D.
Editor

Lissy F. Jarvik, M.D., Ph.D.
Jeffrey R. Foster, M.D.
Jonathan D. Lieff, M.D.
Steven R. Mershon, M.D.
Editorial Committee

This publication was supported by the American Association for Geriatric Psychiatry

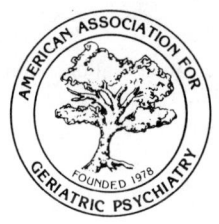

Springer Publishing Company • New York

Copyright © 1988 by Springer Publishing Company, Inc.

All rights reserved

No part of this publication may be reproduced, stored in a retrieval system, or transmitted in any form or by any means, electronic, mechanical, photocopying, recording, or otherwise, without the prior permission of Springer Publishing Company, Inc.

Springer Publishing Company, Inc.
536 Broadway
New York, NY 10012

88 89 90 91 92 / 5 4 3 2 1

LIBRARY OF CONGRESS
Library of Congress Cataloging-in-Publication Data

Essentials of geriatric psychiatry : a guide for health professionals
   / Editorial Committee, American Association for Geriatric Psychiatry
   ; Lawrence W. Lazarus, editor . . . [et al.].
      p. cm.
   Includes bibliographies and index.
   ISBN 0-8261-5990-7
   1. Geriatric psychiatry. I. Lazarus, Lawrence W., 1941-
II. American Association for Geriatric Psychiatry. Editorial
Committee.
      [DNLM: 1. Geriatric Psychiatry. 2. Mental Disorders—in old age.
WT 150 E78]
RC451.4.A5E77 1988
618.97'689—dc 19
DNLM/DLC
for Library of Congress   86-4919
                                                                      CIP

Printed in the United States of America

This publication was supported by an educational grant from the National Institute of Mental Health.

Contents

The American Association for Geriatric Psychiatry	vii
Foreword by Elliott M. Stein	ix
Contributors	xi
1 Normal Aging—Psychological and Sociocultural Aspects *Elliott M. Stein*	1
2 Normal Aging—Biological Aspects *Jeffrey R. Foster*	25
3 Sexuality and Sexual Dysfunction in the Elderly *Eugene M. Dagon*	41
4 Medical Aspects of Aging *Raymond Vickers*	65
5 Principles of Diagnosis and Treatment in Geriatric Psychiatry *James E. Spar*	102
6 Functional Psychiatric Disorders in the Elderly *Ira R. Katz, Sharon Curlik, and Paul Nemetz*	113
7 Alzheimer's Disease and Related Disorders *Jeffrey R. Foster*	138
8 Psychotherapy with the Elderly *Lawrence W. Lazarus and Joel Sadavoy*	147

9   Somatic Therapies in Geriatric Psychiatry   173
   Charles Shamoian

10   The Organization of Mental Health Services   189
   for the Elderly
   The Interuniversity Consortium of Academic GeroPsychiatrists

11   Legal Issues in Geriatric Psychiatry   214
   F. M. Baker and Sanford I. Finkel

12   Financial Issues Affecting Geriatric Psychiatric Care   230
   Gary L. Gottlieb

Index   249

The American Association for Geriatric Psychiatry

The American Association for Geriatric Psychiatry (AAGP) was founded in 1978 by Sanford Finkel, M.D. in response to the growing number of psychiatrists interested in the mental and emotional needs of older people. In its relatively short history, the AAGP has grown to almost 1,000 members in the United States, Canada, and abroad, reflecting the significant expansion of activity in geriatric psychiatry. Members include the psychiatric clinicians, educators, researchers, and administrators who have been in the forefront of an important evolutionary process in medicine, mental health, and the sociocultural milieu of today and tomorrow.

The major goal of the AAGP is to improve the care of patients—those older individuals with mental or emotional disorders. The AAGP has identified four major functional areas in which it works for its members:

1. *Educational*: Members are kept informed of the most recent research developments and other current developments regarding the nature and treatment of the psychiatric disorders of late life. The AAGP sponsors educational programs and written materials for psychiatrists, other health professionals, and the public on topics concerning the mental health and illness of the elderly. The AAGP encourages increased inclusion of, and focus on, geriatrics in psychiatric and other training programs.

2. *Informational*: Members are informed of changes in professional, social, economic, and political events that impact on the practice of geriatric psychiatry.

3. *Interactional*: The AAGP provides a communications network for members, provides a forum and focus for psychiatrists with a shared interest in geriatrics, and encourages increased interaction among those involved in this field for mutual benefit and support.

4. *Representational*: The AAGP serves an advocacy function for geriatric psychiatry; maintains active formal affiliations with the American Psychiatric Association, the National Council on Aging, the International Psychogeriatric Association, and other organizations; and helps to assure that academia, other medical groups, and government organizations are informed of the needs of our patients and our field.

The number and types of activities are continuing to expand through the efforts of many dedicated individuals who have volunteered to aid in this work. The AAGP currently sponsors four to five highly successful and well-received scientific symposia each year at such gatherings as the annual meetings of the American Psychiatric Association, the Gerontological Society of America, the American Society on Aging, the National Council on Aging, the American Geriatrics Society, and the Congress of the International Psychogeriatric Association. The bimonthly AAGP newsletter contains informational articles, literature abstracts, debates, bibliographies, book reviews, summaries, and notices of scientific meetings. The AAGP biographical membership directory has been a valuable tool in creating an interactional network among geriatric clinicians, academicians, and researchers by providing access to others in the field for consultation, information, and referrals. Other ongoing projects include creating a series of patient information brochures, increasing the number of local and regional geriatric psychiatric organizations and meetings, and encouraging more public and governmental awareness of the mental and emotional problems of older people.

Foreword

Expanding upon our past educational efforts, the AAGP, under the leadership of Drs. Alvin Levinson (president, 1982-1984) and Lissy Jarvik (president, 1984-1985), initiated and carried forward the project that has culminated in this book. This book was written for practicing psychiatrists, geriatric psychiatry training programs, primary-care physicians, and other health care professionals wishing to augment their knowledge about geriatric psychiatry. As the title, *Essentials of Geriatric Psychiatry: A Guide for Health Professionals*, implies, the book attempts to capture the essence of the present state of knowledge in the field. The AAGP's goal is to have this book serve as a study and teaching guide for health care professionals. To achieve brevity for the busy clinician and to avoid duplication of currently available larger textbooks, this book was written in an outline-informational style for easy reading. Each chapter contains an extensive reference list for those wishing to pursue particular topics in greater depth.

The beginning chapters discuss normal aging from psychological, sociocultural, and biological perspectives. Sexuality and sexual dysfunction with aging and medical aspects of aging are then summarized, followed by a chapter on principles of diagnosis and treatment in geriatric psychiatry. A chapter on the functional psychiatric disorders is followed by chapters on Alzheimer's disease and related disorders, psychotherapy, and then a review of the somatic therapies.

Models of comprehensive mental health programs for older adults that have practical applications for health professionals involved in planning and administering similar programs are described. The final two chapters summarize legal and financial issues affecting the care of the elderly psychiatric patient—an area of increasing importance in the nation's rapidly changing health care system.

We hope this volume will help provide those involved in geriatric psychiatry, or those interested in aging, with a format for assessing their knowledge and will point out directions for acquisition of new information and understanding.

On behalf of the American Association for Geriatric Psychiatry, I would like to express my sincere appreciation to all those who labored long and hard researching, preparing, writing, and editing this volume, spending their own time and resources for no reason other than their dedication to the field, to their colleagues, and to their patients. Most especially, I would like to thank Lawrence Lazarus, M.D., Chairman of this book's Editorial Committee; Lissy Jarvik, M.D., Ph.D., Consulting Editor; and members of the Editorial Committee—Jeffrey Foster, M.D., Jonathan Lieff, M.D., Steven Mershon, M.D., and the editing assistance of Benjamin Liptzin, M.D.—for their continuing efforts and long hours devoted to bringing this project to completion; Gene Cohen, M.D., Ph.D., for his encouragement and support; Alvin Levinson, M.D., for the inspiration and drive that started it all; Springer Publishing Company for excellent editing suggestions; and all of the past and present officers and board members of AAGP who have worked to promote this effort and all of the projects of AAGP.

ELLIOTT M. STEIN, M.D.
President, American Association
for Geriatric Psychiatry, 1985–1987
January 1988

Contributors

George Alexopoulos, M.D.
Associate Professor of Psychiatry
Cornell University Medical College
New York, New York

F. M. Baker, M.D., M.P.H.
Associate Professor of Psychiatry
University of Texas Health Science
  Center at San Antonio
San Antonio, Texas

John Barsa, M.D.
Director of Geriatric Psychiatry
Vanderbilt Center at Columbia
  Presbyterian Medical Center
New York, New York

Peter Birkett, M.D.
Medical Director
Riverside Nursing Home
Haverstraw, New York

Carl Cohen, M.D.
Director of Geriatric Psychiatry
Downstate Medical Center
Brooklyn, New York

John Copeland, M.A., F.R.C.P., F.R.C. Psych
Director, Institute of Human Aging
Royal Liverpool Hospital
Liverpool, England

Sharon Curlik, D.O.
Instructor, Division of Geriatric
  Psychiatry
Medical College of Pennsylvania
Philadelphia, Pennsylvania

Eugene M. Dagon, M.D.
Associate Professor of Psychiatry
University of South Florida
Tampa, Florida

Sanford I. Finkel, M.D.
Clinical Associate Professor
  of Psychiatry
Northwestern University
Chicago, Illinois

Barry Fogel, M.D.
Director of Psychiatric Medical
  Program
Rhode Island Hospital
Providence, Rhode Island

Jeffrey R. Foster, M.D.
Director of Geriatric Services
  and Training Program
Department of Psychiatry
New York University Medical
  Center
New York, New York

Gary L. Gottlieb, M.D., M.B.A.
Assistant Professor of Psychiatry
University of Pennsylvania
Philadelphia, Pennsylvania

Lois Grau, Ph.D.
Associate Director of Brookdale
  Research Institute on Aging
Fordham University
New York, New York

Barry Gurland, F.R.C. Psych, F.R.C.P.
Director of Center for Geriatrics
Columbia University
and New York State Office of
  Mental Health
New York, New York

Ira R. Katz, M.D., Ph.D.
Associate Professor, Division
  of Geriatric Psychiatry
Medical College of Pennsylvania
Philadelphia, Pennsylvania

Lawrence W. Lazarus, M.D.
Assistant Professor of Psychiatry
Rush Medical College
Chicago, Illinois

Barry Meyers, M.D.
Director, Geriatric Specialty Clinic
New York Hospital
Cornell University Medical Center
New York, New York

Abraham Monk, Ph.D.
Director, Brookdale Institute
  on Aging
Columbia University
New York, New York

Anthony Mustille, M.D.
Executive Director
Willard Psychiatric Center
Willard, New York

Paul Nemetz, M.D.
Professor of Psychiatry
Medical College of Pennsylvania
Philadelphia, Pennsylvania

Joel Sadavoy, M.D.
Head, Department of Psychiatry
Baycrest Centre for Geriatric Care
Toronto, Ontario, Canada

Charles A. Shamoian, M.D., Ph.D.
Professor of Clinical Psychiatry
Cornell University Medical College
New York, New York

James E. Spar, M.D.
Assistant Professor of Psychiatry
School of Medicine
University of California, Los Angeles
Los Angeles, California

Elliott M. Stein, M.D.
President
American Association for Geriatric
  Psychiatry, 1985-1987
Private Practice
Miami Beach, Florida

John Toner, Ed.D.
Co-Director of Fellowship Programs
  at Center for Geriatrics
Columbia University
and New York State Office of
  Mental Health
New York, New York

Raymond Vickers, M.D.
Associate Professor
Department of Family Practice
Upstate Health Sciences Center
Binghamton, New York

1
Normal Aging—Psychological and Sociocultural Aspects

Elliott M. Stein

In this chapter, I will review social and cultural aspects of aging in the United States of the 1980s. This will include discussion of some societal norms; myths about aging; family and marital relationships; and statistics concerning the financial, political, housing, educational, and health status of older people, including sexual and racial factors. Also discussed will be theories of normal intellectual functioning, personality development, and other related aspects of later life.

I. Historical Perspective
(Finkel, Stein, Miller, Cameron, Hontela, and Eisdorfer, 1982)

A. In past centuries, when few people lived to an advanced age and when educational opportunities were comparatively restricted, the older person was viewed as special, successful, and a source of wisdom.

B. In preindustrialized eras, especially in rural/agrarian locations, older people were more likely to own property and were, therefore, at the apex of the hierarchical economic network. With the advent of industrialization, the younger individual could obtain financial independence, while retirement from industrial work caused financial dependence of older persons.

C. Retirement, that is, an unemployed time in the later period of life not brought about by an inability to work, is a relatively new concept.

1. In 1883, Bismarck introduced the idea of mandatory retirement, arbitrarily choosing age 65 as the retirement age. In the 1880s, only 2% of the population was over age 65.
2. Retirement was then and is still promoted as a reward, a permanent vacation, for the long-term worker. These expectations, however, often remain unmet, since the retired individual frequently faces reduced income, loss of status, disruption of interpersonal relationships, isolation, boredom, and identity confusion.
3. Currently, the first 20 years (or more) of an individual's life are usually devoted to education and the time after age 60–65 to retirement. With a life expectancy of 79 years for men of age 65, and nearly 84 years for women of age 65 (as of 1980), this amounts to over 14 and 19 years of retirement, respectively (Heinz, 1984). Therefore, generally only the middle 40 years, less than one-half the lifespan, tend to be spent generating the income that must support those below age 20 and those over age 65.
D. Increased mobility, divorce, and other factors have led to what some believe to be the disintegration of the extended family. While it is true that in past generations families lived together more often than they do now, sometimes because of financial necessity rather than affectionate bonding, the vast majority of older people still maintain frequent contacts with their grown children; many live nearby and participate in intergenerational social interactions, assistance, and celebrations.

II. Current Social and Cultural Aspects of Normal Aging in the United States
(Taeuber, 1983)

A. Stereotypes and Myths (see Figure 1.1)
1. Adults younger than 65 years of age have a different view of what later life is like than older people have of the life they are experiencing. Negative stereotypes held by younger people about the elderly often lead them to overlook positive aspects of aging and to deny and avoid contemplating their own inevitable aging process.
2. Many older people still believe in ageist myths and stereotypes.
3. Little distinction is made by the general population between those groups that have at times been called the young-old (ages 55–75), the middle-old (ages 75–85), and the very-old (over age

Normal Aging—Psychological and Sociocultural Aspects

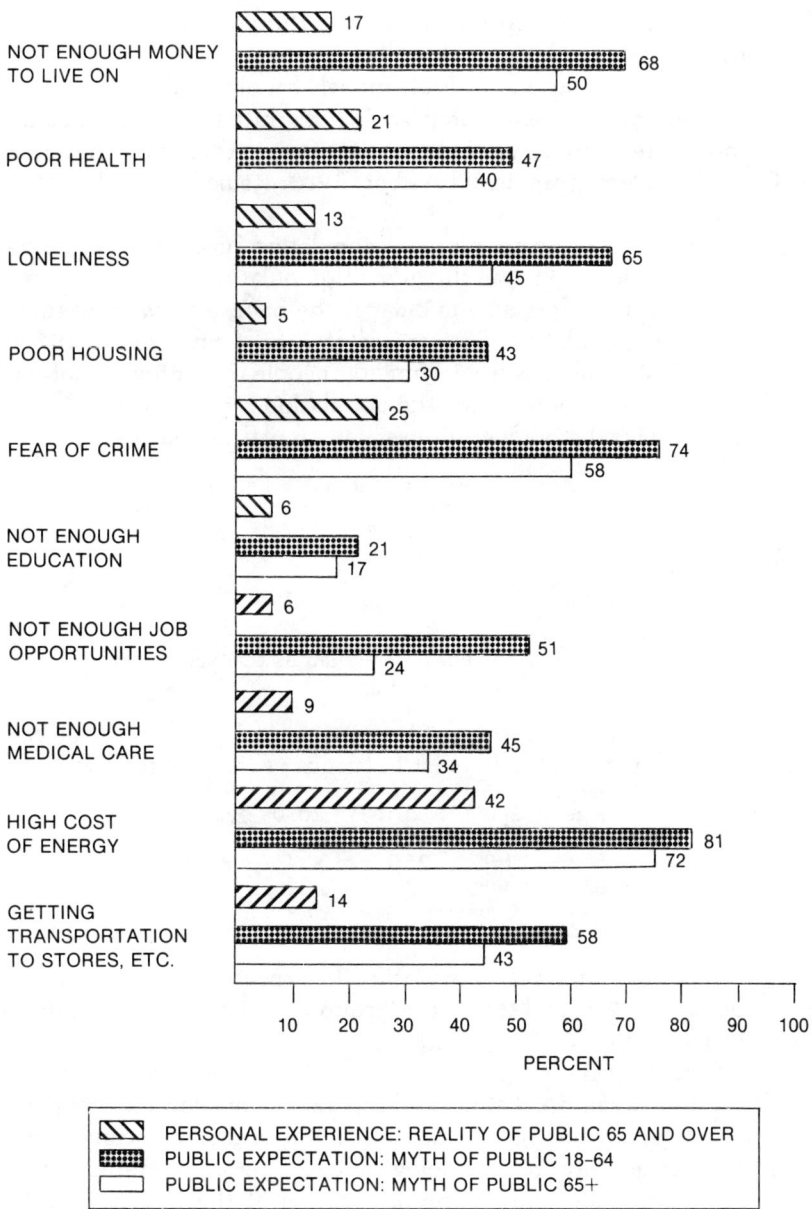

FIGURE 1.1 Myth vs. reality of aging (percent of elderly respondents reporting problems to be very serious vs. the public's expectations of the seriousness of these problems).

Source: Heinz, 1984

85). Some of the differences among these groups are indicated by studies cited later in this chapter.
    4. Positive expectations and role models for older people have been infrequent and inconsistently demonstrated. The few positive models tend to be viewed as exceptions rather than the norm.
B. Changing Demographics (Taeuber, 1983; Redick & Taube, 1980; Heinz, 1986a)
    1. Over the past two decades, the population aged 65 and older has grown twice as fast as the general population.
        a. The group aged 85 and older is the fastest-growing segment of the population: an increase of 165% from 1960 to 1982.
        b. In 1900, there were 3.1 million people over 65 years of age, comprising only 4% of the population.
        c. In 1984, the population breakdown was as follows:

Age	Number (millions)	Percentage
55–65	22.21	9.4
65–74	16.60	7.0
75–84	8.79	3.7
85+	2.50*	1.1

*This includes more than 32,000 people over 100 years of age.

    2. Future projections: the percentage of total population for each age group projected to exist in future years is as follows:

Age	2000	2010	2030	2050
55+	21.9%	26.1%	32.4%	33.9%
65+	13.0%	13.8%	21.2%	21.8%
85+	1.8%	2.3%	2.8%	5.2%

While the total U.S. population is expected to grow by 33% between 1982 and 2050, the group over age 55 is expected to grow 113%.
C. Age Stratification
    Older individuals are distinct and separable from younger people on the basis of various social, functional, physical, and socioeconomic factors, in addition to chronological age. These factors may naturally or artificially inhibit the integration of the elderly with the general population.
    1. Chronological Age
        a. Young-old, old-old (Neugarten, 1977). The young-old are defined as those in postretirement who maintain physical vigor and have new time for leisure and involvement in social, educational, and recreational activities. They may develop

more acute medical problems. Young-old usually refers to people between the ages of 55 and 75. Old-old (or "frail old"), initially used for those over age 75, is now used variously to refer to those aged 75 to 85, with those over 85 being called the very-old. Alternatively, the group aged 65 or 70 to 80 is sometimes called the middle-old. The old-old have a much higher percentage of people who have chronic medical problems or who are more dependent on others for aid of various kinds. Paradoxically, relatively more of these people may be alone (Heinz, 1986a).
   b. Cohort effect is defined as the effect on an individual of having lived through the same historical period. Unique common past experiences draw people together; for example, immigration, wars, and depression.
2. Work Roles
   a. The prestige of employment. The employed individual incorporates his or her job description as a vital portion of self-image and tends to be identified by others in similar terms.
   b. Frequently, the transition from the work role to retirement is made abruptly, without adequate planning or preparation. It may even be involuntary, as in the case of mandatory retirement programs.
   c. Behaviors and prerogatives for the retiree that can serve as substitutes for the work role are poorly defined, as exemplified by the vague terms *leisure role* and *retired person*. The person in the process of retiring may be unaware of specific activities and opportunities available.
3. Social Norms
   a. Stereotypic and prejudicial expectations by the younger population (and, to some extent, the older) may limit the behaviors in which older individuals engage. This is akin to a child's denial that his or her parents have sexual relations and to the old proverb, "You can't teach an old dog new tricks." Older people may also be confronted by changing cultural values, which challenge or alter longstanding opinions, mores, or habits. Conversely, previous outlets for pleasure and maintenance of self-esteem may be less or no longer available.
   b. Reduced prestige of the elderly as a group. The general view of Western culture has not valued the elderly as being productive contributors to society.
   c. Isolation of the elderly from interaction with other age groups. This is exemplified by the removal of older people from the workplace by retirement and the establishment of age-segregated housing.

4. Physical and geographical mobility decreases with advanced age.
   a. Due to reduced income.
   b. Due to impaired health.
   c. Due to limited mobility (26% of those 85 years of age or older need help in walking or traveling outside of the home) (Heinz, 1984).
5. Certain social institutions maintain age stratification.
   a. Retirement.
   b. Tax exemptions; Social Security; Medicare; special nutritional, recreational, and transportation programs.
   c. Private pension plans, senior citizen discounts for older consumers.
   d. Dependency of the aged on these structures has been accepted as a societal norm.

D. Family Relations
  1. Marital Status (Taeuber, 1983)
     a. Because life expectancy for women is considerably greater than that for men, elderly women currently outnumber men 3 to 2 (compared to 1960, when women outnumbered men by only 5 to 4); this is creating a "female gerontocracy" (Somers, 1985). In 1982, there were 80 men aged 65 to 69 for every 100 women, and only 42 men for every 100 women in the group aged 85 and over.
     b. In 1983, living arrangements and marital status differed sharply between men and women over the age of 65 (Heinz, 1986a).
        (1) From ages 65 to 74, 79% of men live with spouses, compared to 49% of women; 7% of men live in households with someone not a spouse, compared to 15% of women; 12% of men live alone, compared to 36% of women; 2% of men and 1% of women live in nonhousehold (i.e., not an independent house or apartment) environments.
        (2) Over the age of 75, 66% of men live with spouses, 8% live in households with nonspouses, and 19% live alone. Of women over the age of 75, 22% live with spouses, 24% live in nonspouse households, and 42% live alone. Eight percent of men and 13% of women over 75 years of age live in nonhousehold environments.
        (3) Between ages 65 and 74, 79% of men were married and living with their spouses, 5% were single, 2% were separated, 9% widowed, and 4% divorced. In the same age range, 49% of women were married and living with their

spouses, 5% were single, 2% separated, 39% widowed, and 5% divorced.
(4) Over the age of 75, 66% of men were married and living with their spouses, 4% single, 3% separated, 24% widowed, and 2% divorced. For women over the age of 75, 22% were married and living with their spouses, 6% single, 1% separated, 67% widowed, and 3% divorced.
(5) Elderly widowed men have remarriage rates 7 times higher than widowed women. The mean duration of widowhood is 6.6 years for men versus 14.3 years for women.
(6) Elderly white males have the highest probability of being married; elderly black females have the lowest.
2. Relations with Children (Bengtson & Treas, 1980; Shanas et al., 1968)
   a. Multigenerational households were more common in past generations. Before Social Security and old-age benefits (1935), kinship groups were the primary resource against the vicissitudes of later life, such as disability, widowhood, and unemployment. Nonetheless, multigenerational households were not the norm then either, primarily because of high death rates and social custom.
   b. Most older people—single, married, or widowed—prefer to live in their own homes in close proximity to, rather than with, their children. The majority live less than 30 miles from at least one of their children (Shanas et al.,1968).
   c. Similarly, there tends to be a high degree of interaction between generations, such as visits, telephone contacts, and so forth.
      (1) In a 1975 survey, only 1 in 10 older Americans reported that he or she had not seen one of his or her children in the past 30 days (Heinz, 1984). In a 1962 three-nation survey (USA, Great Britain, Denmark), of those in the American portion of the sample who lived apart from their children, 52% reported seeing one of the children in the past 1 to 2 days.
   d. Affectional relations appear to be well maintained for the majority of older people, both toward and from their children.
   e. Intergenerational support and assistance (Bengtson & Treas, 1980).
      (1) Moral support and advice.

(2) Exchange of assistance/services—helping and being helped (e.g., shopping, care of grandchildren, provision of shelter).
    (a) Older people are as often the donors as the recipients of help.
(3) Informal activities (recreation, conversation, planning).
(4) Ceremonial or family ritual activities.
(5) Financial assistance.

E. Parent Care (Brody, 1985)
  1. As parents live longer, long-term parent care has become a more normative but stressful process. Instead of the formal system, families (most often adult daughters) provide 80% to 90% of medically related and personal care, household tasks, transportation and shopping, and so forth.
  2. Three-generation and four-generation families are common: about half of all persons aged 65 and older have great-grandchildren (Heinz, 1984).
  3. Financial hardship can be a substantial problem with parent care. However, serious consequences are related to the emotional strain affecting the caregiver's family as well as the primary caregiver.
  4. Adult children must permit aging parents to be dependent, and aging parents must be capable of being dependent. Old family conflicts may surface and increase conflicts in the adult child's "new family." Most family caregivers feel some guilt about not doing enough. They are not able to care for their parents the way their parents cared for them when they were children. Anger and resentment may occur in both parents and children.
  5. For many women, parent care is not a single, time-limited affair, but rather a part of "careers" in caregiving (e.g., for children, parents-in-law, other relatives). They may be encouraged or feel obligated to reduce or entirely give up outside work.
  6. Grandparenthood plays a role.
     a. There is a special relationship between children and grandparents, qualitatively different from the one between children and parents.
     b. Grandparenthood provides a historical perspective on life, family life, and tradition that can be transmitted to the young, thus providing the grandparent with a sense of continuity to his or her life.
     c. Currently, many older people have surviving parents. In 1980, 40% of people in their late fifties, 20% of those in their early sixties, 10% of those in their late sixties, and 3% of those in their seventies had a surviving parent (Brody, 1985).

7. Other familial and nonfamilial support systems exist.
   a. Siblings, cousins, in-laws, and other "peer" relative relationships gain added importance when other relationships are lost and the older person's dependence increases.
   b. Nonkinship, friendship support systems develop and gain increasing importance as spouses and other relatives die or otherwise become less available (due to illness, distance, etc). Dependence upon social service networks and professional caregivers may also increase.
   c. Social networks, as used here, refer to all of an individual's social contacts that provide some emotional or material support. One study (Lubben, 1984) of the elderly has found a strong relationship between the degree of contact with members of a social network and psychological well-being, intellectual functioning, and maintaining activities of daily living.
F. Intellectual Functioning (Botwinick, 1977; Jarvik & Bank, 1983)
   1. Cross-sectional and longitudinal investigations have concluded that increasing adult age brings about some intellectual decline. However, different intellectual functions change with age in different ways.
   2. Up to age 50, and even beyond, there is little or no decrement in cognitive functions using information and skills already achieved, provided speed of response is not a factor. With increasing age, there is a decrease in memory, perceptual-integrative abilities, and on speed tests, especially on nonverbal tests. In many areas, age decline begins around the middle or late forties, although some areas of intellectual functioning show decline in early adulthood. However, one major longitudinal study concluded that there is a general stability of nonspeeded cognitive performance to age 75 and perhaps even older.
   3. Giving older people additional time to respond in test situations improves their test performance but does not eliminate age differences (Botwinick, 1977). There may be an age-related difficulty in retrieving stored information (Arenberg & Robertson-Tchabo, 1977).
   4. Cross-sectional and longitudinal studies suggest that people who perform relatively well when young will also perform relatively well when old. Those who can least afford a loss of intellectual abilities tend to have greater declines than those who were initially more able.
   5. Certain test performance levels or changes in these levels over time apparently relate to the last phase of life or closeness of

death. This "terminal-drop" hypothesis is based on findings that those elderly who perform poorly on intellectual tasks, or who show a decline from former levels, tend to die sooner than those who maintain their intellectual abilities.
G. Personality (Neugarten, 1977)
  1. There are various theories on changes in personality associated with aging.
     a. The last two of Erik Erikson's eight stages of the life cycle
        (1) The crisis of generativity (middle years)—the resolution of this phase involves the development of a concern for future generations and an emotional investment in the products of one's own creation.
        (2) The crisis of ego integrity (late adulthood)—this stage involves developing the sense that life has been the product of one's own making. Failure to maintain integrity results in despair and disgust.
     b. Social-psychological theory
        (1) Personality is the integration of socialization experiences and reactions to social roles.
        (2) Personality is not a stable internal entity but is continually changing in response to environmental, social, and historical influences.
     c. Cognitive theory
        (1) Central concepts of this theory are: perception of others, perceived situation, and perceived self are more related to behavior change than are actual objective changes. Individual personality differences are influenced by differing perceptions.
        (2) The aging personality should not be defined in terms of stable traits, but in terms of changing cognitive perceptions.
H. Other Aspects of Age-Related Changes with Aging
  1. Since people age at different rates in the biopsychosocial spheres, there is a need to distinguish between chronological, social, biological, and psychological aging. Perceptions of age may vary by age, sex, and social class. For example, for an upper-middle-class person, middle age may represent the prime of life; for a blue-collar worker, it may signal slowing down and physical weakening.
  2. Distance from death assumes greater importance with advancing years, compared with chronological age (i.e., distance from birth).
  3. Several studies have found that introversion increases with age in the second half of life. Role activity decreases. Disengagement

theory (Cumming & Henry, 1961) holds that the decreased social interaction in old age is a result of both societal and individual withdrawal, along with decreased emotional involvement in various activities and relationships. Some evidence suggests that disengagement as a process of aging is not the norm but is a response to the loss of traditional culture (Gutmann, 1977). Activity theory may be seen as the opposite of disengagement theory, postulating that active involvement is conducive to "successful" aging.
4. No age-related differences are found in goal-directed and purposeful behavior, coping styles, satisfaction with life, or those processes more readily available to conscious control. There are individual differences that are maintained over time (Neugarten, 1977).
5. Sex differences exist. Older men appear more receptive than younger men to their affiliative, nurturant, and sensual promptings; older women, to their aggressive and egocentric impulses (Neugarten, 1977).
6. Some important events and issues in old age include: menopause (women) and the empty-nest syndrome (departure of grown children), retirement, time left to live, the personalization of death, the rehearsal for widowhood (women), the rehearsal for illness, the loss of significant others, concerns about disability and dependency, the yielding of a sense of competency and authority, integrity (the importance of what one has been rather than what one is), the heritage one leaves behind, and putting one's memories into order. It is not necessarily the event itself, but how prepared an individual is for it, that determines the effects of the event or issue on the personality.
7. Paranoia may have some adaptive value in the elderly—grouchiness and suspiciousness may have some survival value in old age, as, for example, in the nursing home setting.
8. Common sense dictates that cohort factors influence personality—different cohorts have experienced different social events and consequently may perform differently on personality measures.

I. Cross-Cultural Studies (Gutmann, 1977)
1. Cross-cultural studies have noted that societies that encourage an egocentric attitude tend, in general, to be harshest in their treatment of the elderly (e.g., in the Ammassalik Eskimos of Greenland, power and possession are very important, murder at any age goes unpunished, and the elderly are sometimes left to die in the cold when they can no longer provide for them-

selves). In contrast, societies that encourage altruism provide more security for their elderly (e.g., in the Nunivak Eskimos of the Bering Sea, warm kinship ties extend to, and protect, the elderly).
2. In many cultures, there seems to be an evolution in males, as they progress from middle-age to old age, from active mastery to passive mastery. For example, in Oriental cultures young men are expected to work hard to achieve in the pragmatic world, while older men are expected to focus on religious aspirations. In addition, across some cultures, older men tend to become more interested in values, interests, and activities that are no longer stereotypically masculine.
3. In many cultures there seems to be the opposite movement: as women move from middle age to old age, they move from passive to active mastery. For example, in Amerindian and Mexican cultures postmenopausal Amerindians are generally given more sexual freedom and are allowed to participate in ritual and healing practices. Older Mexican-American women are considered very important and powerful in the home.

J. Sex, Race, and Class Differences in Aging
  1. Some Sex Differences
     a. The rate of remarrying for widowers is eight times higher than that for widows.
     b. Over 45% of single, divorced, or widowed women live below the poverty level, compared to 33% of men.
     c. Despite a longer life expectancy, women between the ages of 60 and 94 tend to rate their health as worse than men who are in the same age group.
     d. Older women are more active in religious and community organizations than older men.
  2. Some Socioeconomic Differences
     a. Contact with family, friends, and neighbors seems to be more frequent among elderly with higher socioeconomic status, although working-class elderly receive more actual assistance from their children (e.g., living in the same household and receiving actual, hands-on assistance).
     b. Elderly of upper socioeconomic status tend to be more involved in community activities than elderly of lower socioeconomic status.
  3. Some Ethnic Differences
     a. Minority aged have a reduced longevity until they reach ages above 65 (Heinz, 1986b). After age 65, some minority groups tend to live longer.

	Life expectancy (in years)	
	At age 65	At age 80
Black men	0.5	9.1
White men	6.8	6.9
Black women	8.7	11.9
White women	13.8	9.2

b. Minority elderly are far more likely to be poor and are more likely to retire because of poor physical health (Heinz, 1986a).

	Percentage of population over age 65 below poverty level (1983)
Blacks	36.3%
Whites	12.0%
Hispanics	23.1%

	Percentage of population retired due to poor health (Southern California; Bengtson, Kasschau, & Ragen, 1977)
Blacks	55%
Mexican-Americans	49%
Whites	27%

c. In one major southern California study comparing elderly Mexican-Americans, blacks, and Anglos, Mexican-Americans had the lowest rate of interaction with friends and neighbors, Anglos the highest. Yet Anglos had less interaction with their families and relatives than either blacks or Mexican-Americans (Bengtson et al., 1977).

d. There is some indication that the black aged have higher participation in community and political organizations than Anglos (when socioeconomic status is held constant).

e. Since the above ethnic comparisons in a–d are derived from a limited number of isolated studies, futher research is needed.

K. Political and Community Activities
  1. Older people tend to have the highest percentage of voter participation of any age group. In November 1980, when the rate for the general population (25 and over) was 59.2%, the voter participation for persons 55 to 64 years of age was 71%, for those 65 to 74 years of age it was 69%, and for those 75 years of age and older it was 58%.
  2. Older people today are organizing more into age-oriented self-help, activist, and political groups.

3. Many volunteer activities in communities are performed by older persons.
4. Second and third careers and participation in continuing education programs, altruistic activities, and advisory roles are increasingly common among the elderly.

L. Religion (Heinz, 1984)
  1. Elderly persons have the highest rate of religiosity of all age groups.
  2. As age increases, so do the following measures of spiritual commitment: the influence of religion in life; putting religious beliefs into practice; and degree of personal comfort and support from religion.

M. Education (Heinz, 1984, 1986a)
  1. The median educational attainment of people over age 65 is well below that of those under 65, but it is increasing.
     a. In 1970, the median years of school completed by those over 65 was 8.7 years, compared to 12.2 years for the entire population. By 1983, the median years of school completed by those over 65 had increased to 11.0 years, compared to 12.5 median years for the entire population.
     b. In 1981, 10.9% of all adult education students were 65 years of age or older.

N. Economic Issues (Taeuber, 1983)
  1. The elderly are characterized by lower and less secure incomes, compared to the general population and compared to the elderly themselves when they were younger. Incomes and sources of support, social services, and community resources are not currently increasing at the same rate as the elderly population is increasing.
  2. Lower income may be associated with factors over which the individual may have little or no control: sex, race, health status, and survival of spouse or self. Current income among the elderly may depend on past educational achievement, lifetime earnings and investments, age of retirement, and economic and political conditions of locality and country.
  3. In 1984 the following statistics applied (Heinz, 1986b; Taeuber, 1983):
     a.

Age (years)	Median income of families	Single individuals
25–64	$28,972	$15,028
65+	18,118	7,286
85+	13,750	6,223

Normal Aging—Psychological and Sociocultural Aspects

b. The pattern for women alone is similar, but the decline begins at age 50 and income is at much lower levels:

Median income (1984)	
Men 65+	$10,450
Women 65+	$ 6,020

c. Yearly income (Heinz, 1986)—See Figure 1.2.
d. Racial differences (Heinz, 1986a):

Race and sex	Median income 1984 Age 65–69	Age 70+
White men	$12,749	$9,407
Black men	7,545	5,679
Hispanic men	8,778	5,705
White women	6,527	6,225
Black women	4,446	4,304
Hispanic women	4,342	4,825

e. Differences by living status (in those over 65 years of age):

Living status	Median income 1981
Alone	$ 5,154
With family	$14,335

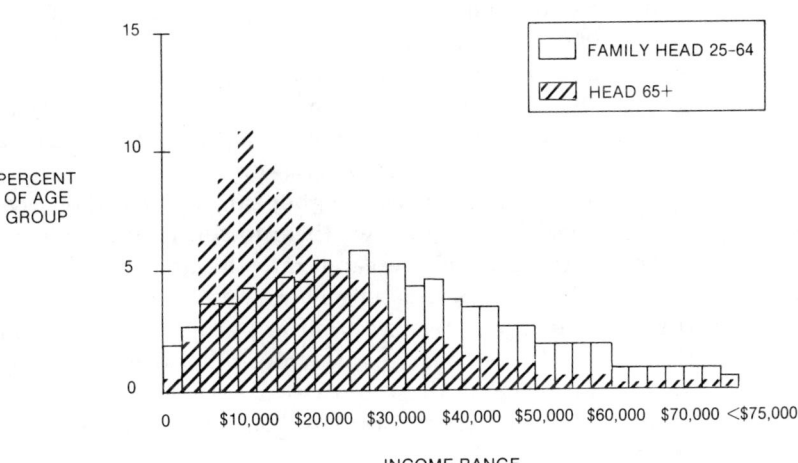

FIGURE 1.2 Distribution of money income of families, elderly and nonelderly, 1984 (from Heinz, 1986b).

4. Sources of Income (Taeuber, 1983)
   a. Social Security is the largest single source of income for the elderly. Social Security is received by 91% of the elderly population, constituting over half of income for over half of this population.
   b. Income sources for the typical elderly person in 1981 were: Social Security, 37%; earnings, 25%; property income (rents, dividends, interest), 23%; and private and public pensions, 13%.
      (1) Over the past 20 years in the United States there has been a decline for the elderly in the importance of earnings and increased reliance on income from Social Security, public and private pensions, and assets.
      (2) Income from Social Security increases in relative importance as a person ages.
      (3) In 1978, most elderly with property income received less than $1,000 a year from that source. Those with pensions received an average of less than $2,000 a year from that source.
      (4) In 1981, only 2% of the elderly relied on pensions for more than half of their incomes.
   c. Current earnings make the greatest difference with regard to the economic well-being of older persons.
      (1) Year-round, full-time workers have incomes close to those of younger people until the age of 70, when median income of full-time workers drops from $19,000 to $16,000. About half of full-time workers over age 65 have incomes between $10,000 and $30,000.
      (2) In 1984, year-round, full-time workers included (Heinz, 1986a): 12.0 million individuals aged 55 to 64 and 2.9 million individuals aged 65 and over.
      (3) It is likely that those with higher earnings are in relatively good health, which allows them to continue working.
   d. There is little available research into the nature and characteristics of people beginning new careers after retiring from their principal job. Similarly, differing orientations toward retirement of blue-collar versus white-collar workers, the sick versus the healthy, those with social options versus those without, and so forth need further assessment in retirement research (Cohen, 1980).
5. Poverty (Taeuber, 1983; Heinz, 1986a)
   a. Many elderly people face poverty for the first time in their lives after retirement.

b. Poverty levels in 1981 were considered to be below $5,498 for elderly families and below $4,359 for elderly individuals. In 1984, the poverty level for a family of four was considered to be below $10,609 and for an elderly couple, below $6,282.
c. Percentage of those over age 65 below poverty level:

Year	Percentage
1959	33%
1970	25%
1981	15.3%
1984	12.4%

d. Poverty levels were highest among the aged, women, minorities, those who lived alone, the unmarried, the unemployed, those who depended exclusively on Social Security benefits, and those who lived in small towns and rural areas.
e. In most states, poverty rates among the aged were slightly higher than the rate for all persons, except for New York, Arizona, California, and Florida. In the latter three states, migration of relatively more affluent retirees may have raised the annual income of these states' elderly. The highest poverty rates in 1979 for the aged were found in Mississippi (34.3%), Alabama (28.2%), and Arkansas (28.2%); the lowest rates were in California (8.3%), Connecticut (8.8%), and Wisconsin (9.6%).
f. Of all poor persons 60 years of age and older, just over half lived in metropolitan areas and the remainder lived in small towns and rural areas. In 1981, the poverty rate for the elderly in metropolitan areas was 11.5%, but in the rural areas it was 18.6%. For aged black women in rural areas, the poverty rate was over 60%.
g. Noncash benefits
   (1) Government definitions of poverty do not include a valuation of public housing, subsidized rentals, or medical care. If the value of these benefits, received by some elderly persons, was regarded as income, the poverty rates noted above would obviously change. Estimating the true poverty levels, taking noncash benefits into consideration, would depend greatly on the methods used and the types of benefits included. For example:
      (a) Including food and housing benefits only reduces the poverty rate for the elderly from 14.7% to 12.9%.

(2) Except for medical care under Medicare, most noncash benefits received by the elderly are "means-tested," that is, income criteria determine the person's eligibility.
   (a) Of the 1.1 million elderly receiving food stamps in 1981, 86% had incomes below 125% of poverty level (that is, less than 25% higher than the poverty level) and received food stamps with a value of less than $500 annually.
   (b) Five percent of the elderly lived in subsidized housing.
   (c) About 2.5 million elderly (14%) received Medicaid benefits, and 16.8 million elderly households had at least one person covered by Medicare.
(3) The persistence of the relatively high rates of poverty among the elderly in spite of relatively high allocations of the federal budget for elderly program recipients seems a paradox. There are at least three explanations for this apparent paradox.
   (a) A large proportion (40%) of the elderly with incomes below the poverty level do not participate in means-tested programs designed to assist them.
   (b) Of the $200 billion spent in the federal budget for the fiscal year 1982 for the elderly, 92% was allocated to retirement and health insurance programs that are largely self-funded by lifetime contributions from individuals and employers. Only $16 billion, or 2.1% of the budget, was spent to assist low-income persons through cash or in-kind means-tested programs.
   (c) The principal means-tested programs, such as Supplemental Security Income, pay maximum benefits that still leave the elderly person below the poverty level.

O. Housing and Environmental Issues (Taeuber, 1983; Heinz, 1986b)
  1. In 1983, 73% of households maintained by elderly people were owner-occupied.
     a. Nearly 80% of these were owned free and clear, according to the 1980 census.
     b. Of all homes owned free and clear, 67% are maintained by an elderly person.
  2. Home ownership is most common in intact families, but 37% of owner-occupied elderly households were inhabited by elderly men and women living alone.
  3. For renter-occupied elderly households, 33% were maintained by elderly persons in families and 67% were maintained by elderly persons living alone.
  4. Most older people remain in the geographic area where they

spent most of their adult lives. Older people moved from one house to another at only 50% the rate of the general population (20% for the elderly vs. 45% for all adults) for the five-year period 1975-1980.
5. Similarly, only 4% of the elderly moved to a different state, compared to 90% of the general population.
   a. There was a net migration from 1970 to 1980 of older people away from the northeast, middle-Atlantic, and north-central states to retirement areas, rural areas, and small towns in the South and West, especially Florida, Texas, Nevada, and California.
      (1) Of the population over 65 who lived in the West in 1980, 7% were new residents since 1975.
      (2) In the South in 1980, 6% of the population over age 65 were new residents since 1975.
      (3) These figures compare with only 2% of new elderly residents in northeast and north-central states during the same time period.
6. Retirement Communities
   These may be complete, architecturally designed, planned retirement communities, or they may be *de facto*, unplanned towns that have attracted large numbers of older residents.
   a. Residents in these areas confront potential problems because of
      (1) Age segregation, with attendant lack of stimulation from younger age groups and stereotyping of, and by, the elderly.
      (2) High competition among the elderly for available community resources and social services, such as: employment, education and volunteer opportunities, housing, senior citizen centers and other senior programs, financial assistance, and medical care.
   b. Geographical dislocation to retirement communities may isolate elderly persons from long-established social/familial support networks and from familiar environments.
7. Crime Victimization (Kasl & Rosenfeld, 1980)
   a. The elderly are less likely to be victims of crime, but certain crimes are overrepresented among the elderly (robbery with injury, larceny with personal contact).
      (1) These are more likely to take place in the elderly person's dwelling than in public places.
   b. Older people are more vulnerable to the impact of crime and their fear can be greater, even though their actual exposure to crime is below average.
   c. Lower rates of victimization may result from defensive maneuvers that restrict their mobility and quality of life.

- d. Surveys have found that older people
    - (1) List "crime in the streets" as one of the two or three most serious problems in their neighborhood.
    - (2) Have greater fear of walking alone at night in some areas of their neighborhood than younger people.
        - (a) This fear is especially prominent in those dwelling alone, those in urban and suburban areas, those with low income, and those with poorer relations with neighbors.
    - (3) Have lower perceptions of the safety of their neighborhoods than younger people.
    - (4) Are less willing to report crimes.
- e. Crimes against the elderly are more common in large urban areas and inner cities than in rural areas.
- f. One study found that 76% of elderly people in one inner-city area had been robbed within a 6-month period (Stein, Linn, Slater, & Stein, 1984).

P. Health Status (Taeuber, 1983)
1. There has been a shift in patterns of illness, coinciding with advances in medical technology and care. At the beginning of this century, the elderly were predominantly confronted with acute medical problems; currently, chronic conditions are the most prevalent health problems for the elderly.
    - a. Over 80% of people over age 65 have at least one chronic medical problem, and multiple conditions are common.
    - b. At the turn of the century, infections and parasitic diseases were the major causes of illness. Now the major causes are chronic diseases, accidents (especially traffic accidents), and stress-related conditions (Omram, 1977).
        - (1) The leading chronic conditions causing limitation of activity for the elderly are arthritis, heart conditions (these two account for half of the total), hypertension without heart involvement, and impairment of the back and spine.
        - (2) Stress-related conditions include hypertension, attempted suicide, and drug dependency.
    - c. The principle diagnoses of the elderly made by doctors in 1980–1981 were hypertension, diabetes, chronic ischemic heart disease, cataracts, and osteoarthritis.
2. Interestingly, older people view themselves as healthier than they are stereotypically assumed to be. In 1980, only 8% of elderly people in a study population said their health was poor (Heinz, 1984).

a. Forty percent reported that a major activity had been limited for health reasons (compared with 20% of the population aged 45 to 64). However, 54% of the elderly reported no limitations of any kind. Not until age 85 do over half the population report limitations in carrying out a major activity because of chronic illness.
b. There is a tendency for subjective evaluation of health status to be somewhat more optimistic than objectively measured health ratings. Similarly, health complaints do not differentiate between older and younger cohorts of older persons, though the older cohort tends to have an objectively determined poorer health status. This tendency to minimize health impairment is attributed to a motivational variable, "aspiration level regarding health," a variable that decreases with increasing age. Thus, the same subjective perception of good health may be expressed to the same degree in more ill aged persons as in less ill younger persons.
c. Many older people report more concern and stress about chronic illness and fears of disability and dependency than about sudden illness and death.
d. Good health is associated with higher incomes: 40% of those with incomes over $25,000 reported excellent health, compared to less than 25% of those with incomes under $7,000.
3. Medical Care
   a. People aged 65 and older utilize medical facilities more frequently than younger people: 6 doctor visits are made by the elderly for every 5 made by the general population.
   b. The elderly are hospitalized approximately twice as often as the younger population, stay twice as long, and use twice as many prescription drugs (these statistics are pre-DRG).
      (1) For the very old (over 85 years), there are 75% more hospitalizations than for the group aged 65 to 74, and the average stay is 12 days, compared to 6 days for those under age 65.
      (2) Since 1965, when Medicare was enacted, elderly people have increased their use of hospitals 50%, compared to an 11% increase for the total population.
   c. Mental health. Estimates from 1976 to 1979 indicate that from 15% to 25% of elderly in the community have symptoms of significant mental illness. Depression occurs in about 10%, and dementia of various etiologies accounts for 5% to 6% of the mental disorders of the elderly.
      (1) Among nursing home residents, about 56% suffer from a

chronic mental condition related to some variety of organic mental disorder.
   (2) The elderly use mental health services at less than half the rate of the general population, 7 versus 16 admissions to a psychiatric unit per 1,000. A major trend in the past decade has been a geographic movement of emotionally impaired older people from large state hospitals to nursing homes and to communities.
  d. About 5% of the elderly population live in nursing homes. In 1982, 1.3 million people lived in nursing homes, including 1.5% of those 65 to 74 years of age (232,000 people), 6% of those 75 to 84 years of age (527,000 people), and 23% of those 85 years of age or older (557,000 people).
   (1) The rate of nursing home use has doubled since the inception of Medicare and Medicaid.
   (2) Seventy-five percent of nursing home residents have no spouse, compared to 40% of the noninstitutionalized.
  e. Mortality statistics for 1983 (Heinz, 1986b)—see Table 1.1.
   (1) Factors that have led to reductions in mortality (e.g., from heart disease and stroke) may or may not also lead to reductions in morbidity.

TABLE 1.1 Ten Leading Causes of Death by Older Age Groups, 1983*†
[Rates per 100,000 Population in Specified Group]

	55–64	65–74	75–84	85+
All causes	1,299	2,883	6,310	15,422
Diseases of heart	467	1,144	2,737	7,503
Malignant neoplasms	439	832	1,228	1,611
Cerebrovascular diseases	59	184	652	1,986
Accidents and adverse effects	36	49	101	268
Chronic obstructive pulmonary disease	45	142	259	303
Pneumonia and influenza	16	48	197	857
Diabetes	25	65	125	195
Suicide	17	17	25	22
Chronic liver/cirrhosis	36	39	34	18
Atherosclerosis	5	18	97	537

(Note: It should be noted that data for causes of death are based on information taken from death certificates and that frequently underlying causes are not listed but a secondary illness will be recorded.)
*Alzheimer's disease, often cited as the fourth leading cause of death among the elderly, has no separate listing.
†The numbers have been rounded.

Source: Monthly Vital Statistics Report, Provisional Data 1983, vol. 32 No. 9, Sept. 21, 1985, table 8.

REFERENCES

Arenberg, O., & Robertson-Tchabo, E. A. (1977). Learning and aging. In J. E. Birren & K. W. Schaie (Eds.), *Handbook of the Psychology of Aging* (pp. 421-449). New York: Van Nostrand Reinhold.

Bengtson, V. L., Kasschau, P. L., & Ragan, P. K. (1977). The impact of social structure on aging individuals. In J. E. Birren & K. W. Schaie (Eds.), *Handbook of the Psychology of Aging* (pp. 327-353). New York: Van Nostrand Reinhold.

Bengtson, V., & Treas, J. (1980). The changing family context of mental health and aging. In J. E. Birren & R. B. Sloane (Eds.), *Handbook of Mental Health and Aging* (pp. 400-428). Englewood Cliffs, NJ: Prentice-Hall.

Botwinick, J. (1977). Intellectual abilities. In J. E. Birren & K. W. Schaie (Eds.), *Handbook of the Psychology of Aging* (pp. 580-603). New York: Van Nostrand Reinhold.

Brody, E. M. (1985). The Donald P. Kent Memorial Lecture. Parent care as a normative family stress. *The Gerontologist*, 25(1), pp. 19-29.

Cohen, G. D. (1980). Prospects for Mental Health and Aging. In J. E. Birren & R. B. Sloane (Eds.), *Handbook of Mental Health and Aging* (pp. 972-976). Englewood Cliffs, NJ: Prentice-Hall.

Cumming, E., & Henry, W. E. (1961). *Growing Old*. New York: Basic Books.

Finkel, S., Stein, E., Miller, N., Cameron, I., Hontela, S., & Eisdorfer, C. (1982). Special perspectives on treatment planning for the elderly. In J. Lewis & G. Usdin (Eds.), *Treatment Planning in Psychiatry* (pp. 377-433). Washington, DC: American Psychiatric Association.

Gutmann, D. (1977). The cross-cultural perspective: Notes toward a comparative psychology of aging. In J. E. Birren & K. W. Schaie (Eds.), *Handbook of the Psychology of Aging* (pp. 302-326). New York: Van Nostrand Reinhold.

Heinz, J., Chair, U.S. Senate Special Committee on Aging. (1984). *Aging America*. Washington, DC: U.S. Government Printing Office.

Heinz, J., Chair, U.S. Senate Special Committee on Aging. (1986a). *Aging America—Trends and Projections, 1985-86*. Washington, DC: U.S. Government Printing Office.

Heinz, J., Chair, U.S. Senate Special Committee on Aging. (1986b). *Developments in aging: 1985* (Vol. 3) (Report 99-242). Washington, DC: U.S. Government Printing Office.

Jarvik, L. F., & Bank, L. (1983). Aging twins: Longitudinal psychometric data. In K. W. Schaie (Ed.), *Longitudinal Studies of Adult Psychological Development* (pp. 40-63). New York: Guilford.

Kasl, S. V., & Rosenfeld, S. (1980). The residential environment and its impact on the mental health of the aged. In J. Birren & R. B. Sloane (Eds.), *Handbook of Mental Health and Aging* (pp. 481-482). Englewood Cliffs, NJ: Prentice-Hall.

Lubben, J. E. (1984, November). *Ethnic and gender differences in the relationship of social networks on the health status of the aged*. Paper presented at the annual meeting of the Gerontological Society of America, San Antonio, Texas.

Neugarten, B. L. (1977). Personality and aging. In J. E. Birren & K. W. Schaie (Eds.), *Handbook of the Psychology of Aging* (pp. 626-649). New York: Van Nostrand Reinhold.

Omram, A. R. (1977, May). *Epidemiological Transition in the United States: Health Factors in Population Change.* [Population bulletin, 32(2)]. Washington, DC: Population Reference Bureau.

Ragan, P., & Wales, J. (1980). Age stratification and the life course. In J. Birren & R. B. Sloane (Eds.), *Handbook of Mental Health and Aging* (pp. 377-399). Englewood Cliffs, NJ: Prentice-Hall.

Redick, R., & Taube, C. (1980). Demography and mental health care of the aged. In J. Birren & R. B. Sloane (Eds.), *Handbook of Mental Health and Aging* (pp. 57-71).) Englewood Cliffs, NJ: Prentice-Hall.

Shanas, E., Townsend, P., Wedderbarn, D., Friis, H., Milhaj, P., & Sterhouwer, J. (1968). *Old People in Three Industrial Societies.* London: Routledge & Kegan Paul.

Somers, A. R. (1985). Toward a female gerontocracy? Current social trends. In M. R. Haug, A. B. Ford, & M. Sheafor (Eds.), *The Physical and Mental Health of Aged Women* (pp. 16-40). New York: Springer.

Stein, S., Linn, M., Slater, E., & Stein, E. (1984). Future life concerns and recent life events in the elderly. *Journal of the American Geriatrics Society, 32*(6), 431-434.

Taeuber, C. M. (1983). *America in Transition: An Aging Society* (U.S. Bureau of the Census, Current Population Reports, Series P-23, No. 128). Washington, DC: U.S. Government Printing Office.

2

Normal Aging— Biological Aspects

Jeffrey R. Foster

INTRODUCTION

Geriatric psychiatry is distinctive in that multiple domains of change may be simultaneously causing or influencing mental disturbances in the elderly. These domains are illustrated in Figure 2.1. In this chapter, I will focus on the category of normal biological changes with aging.

The intent of this overview is to place the psychiatry of older adults in the broader context of multiple biological changes in function that occur with normal aging. An appreciation of the changing normal biological substrate is necessary for understanding and evaluating the emergence of illness (physical and mental) in the senium. Since space restrictions preclude a review of every organ system, a selective approach is used: (1) to highlight those systems where significant age changes in function clearly occur; (2) to emphasize changes that can potentially influence normal mentation and behavior; (3) to document changes that may affect therapeutics; and (4) to correct misconceptions of "normal" aging concerning mental functioning (e.g., intelligence and memory capabilities). The emphasis on functional changes usually precludes discussion of anatomic changes; the reason is that a multitude of anatomic changes do not have clear functional counterparts and would distract from our purpose. For similar reasons, certain physiologic changes are omitted (e.g., EEG slowing), since their functional significance is not clear or it is uncertain if they reflect aging or disease states.

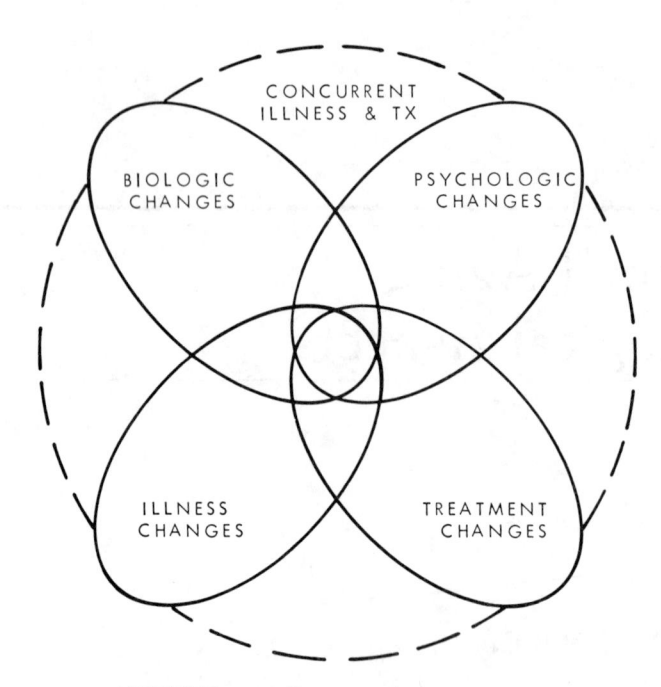

FIGURE 2.1 Geriatric distinctiveness.

Finally, judgments were made that age changes discussed should affect both sexes and should be potentially relevant to psychiatrists regarding their older patients. Thus, for example, the musculoskeletal system (and osteoporosis) as well as the hematopoietic and dermatologic systems were omitted. The immune system is included because of the prevalence of infectious and neoplastic disease in the elderly as well as evidence suggesting that some psychiatric disturbances (e.g., bereavement) may be associated with immune system changes.

A classic problem in gerontology is the differentiation of disease changes from true changes related to the aging process per se. A hallmark of true age-related changes is their gradual evolution over time. These biologic changes often begin subtly in the late twenties, thirties, or forties and continue thereafter; however, they may not reach clinical significance for many years. The direction of adult biological change is usually downward toward lesser degrees of competence or capacity. The rate of change varies substantially with each system or function. Among these systems, the healthy senescent brain holds most of its functional level quite well in absolute terms and relative to decrements in other organ systems. In fact, it is the only organ for which evidence suggests some functional competences may actually increase with aging (e.g., crystallized intelligence).

The overview will be organized as follows: (1) special senses (auditory and visual); (2) central nervous system (learning, memory, intelligence, reaction time); (3) sleep; (4) cardiovascular; (5) pulmonary; (6) endocrine; (7) sexual function; (8) gastrointestinal; (9) renal; (10) immunologic.

I. Changes in Special Senses

A. Auditory Changes (Fisch, 1985; Corso, 1977; Olsho, Harkins, & Lenhardt, 1985)
  1. A gradual age-associated sensorineural impairment evolves from the third decade onward.
  2. About one-third of the population over age 65 suffers from sufficient hearing impairment to have unfavorable social consequences.
  3. Hearing loss is one of the main contributors to the difficulty older people sometimes have in understanding speech. High-frequency sounds are lost first and can lead to difficulties in understanding speech. Vowel sounds are mainly in the lower range, while consonants are in a higher frequency.
  4. Reductions in sound clarity and comprehension may have broader effects than purely sensory loss. Social isolation, depression, and paranoid tendencies may evolve when an older person cannot reliably understand speech.
B. Visual Changes (Fozard, 1977; Kline & Schieber, 1985)
  1. Lens: decreased accommodation for near objects; lens yellowing contributes to need for more illumination; discerning colors at upper spectrum (yellow, orange, red) is better than at lower end (violet, green, blue).
  2. Retinal changes: may be more a reflection of decreased circulation and thus pathologic rather than normal changes; results in further decrease in acuity, color perception, and sensitivity to low levels of illumination.
  3. Age-related changes include reduced visual acuity, reduced capacity to adjust to changes in illumination (dark adaptation), and shift in color vision. These may put older persons at higher risk for falls in lower-illumination settings. Proper lighting and colors may enhance quality of life and functioning in long-term-care facilities.

II. Central Nervous System Changes

A. Learning and Memory Changes (Hultsch & Deutsch, 1981; Schaie & Geiwitz, 1982)
   1. Learning is the acquisition of new information and thus may be considered a part of memory processes. Memory processes include encoding (learning), storage, and retrieval phases.
   2. Encoding (Learning) Phase
      a. Experimental data (mainly cross-sectional) accumulated by psychologists studying learning and memory suggest only slight changes in these functions prior to about age 65, after which there is a rapid decline.
      b. Factors that *reversibly* disadvantage the performance of the elderly include rapid pace (lack of time), poor motivation (caution, anxiety, disinterest), and reduced "depth" of early information processing or use of organizing strategies (e.g., mnemonic or other devices) and impairment of the senses.
   3. Storage phase
      a. The sensory store is a brief (0.25–0.5 sec) representation of pure ("unprocessed") visual or auditory input and decays without further processing; it is regarded as part of the peripheral nervous system input; age-related decrements have been shown, but their significance is uncertain and they are considered to have limited significance to overall age differences in memory performance (Hultsch & Deutsch, 1981).
      b. The short-term store (primary memory) holds a limited amount of information (less than 10 words) for about 10 to 20 seconds. Its purpose is presumably to "work on" the information so it is in proper form for the more permanent long-term store (secondary memory). Although there is evidence that the rate of search through primary memory may decrease with age, the overall capacity of this system appears to be unaffected by age (Hultsch & Deutsch, 1981).
      c. The long-term store (secondary memory) is a permanent maintenance system. Once information has entered secondary memory it is unclear if it is ever forgotten. However, information can be irretrievable on at least a temporary basis. There is conflicting data concerning age changes in long-term memory processes.
         (1) Laboratory testing (e.g., recall vs. recognition of words) suggests distinct longitudinal retrieval deficits over adult life (Schaie & Geiwitz, 1982, pp. 321–323).

(2) Methods testing real-world knowledge show no age-related secondary memory (long-term) changes; also, older adults appear to have no deficits concerning knowledge of their own memory ("metamemory") (Hultsch & Deutsch, 1981, pp. 151-156).
    4. Extensive data suggest that learning and memory function is relatively well preserved until late in life. Learning shows mild age declines. The problem the aged have is in learning new information, procedures, and so forth. Short-term storage remains intact. Data on long-term storage and retrieval problems may represent experimental artifacts or overestimate the degree of normal age-related change. It is difficult to be certain if late-life learning and memory impairment represents true age changes or subclinical disease.
B. Changes in Intelligence (Hultsch & Deutsch, 1981, pp. 97-127; Huyck & Hoyer, 1982, pp. 162-194; Schaie & Geiwitz, 1982, pp. 203-238)
    1. Intelligence usually refers to the capacity for new learning. There are a variety of ways to measure intelligence and different research strategies for assessing change over adulthood (e.g., longitudinal studies, cross-sectional studies, combinations of the two—e.g., cross-sequential studies).
    2. The Wechsler Adult Intelligence Scale (WAIS) has 11 subtests (6 are "verbal"; 5 are "performance"). Often the verbal subtests hold up well with aging, whereas performance subtests show gradual decline.
    3. Initial cross-sectional studies using IQ tests like the WAIS seemed to show clear and progressive declines of scores with age after age 30. Subsequent longitudinal studies of the same people as they actually grew older showed a different picture; that is, that intelligence appears to hold up rather well until late life and that progressive decline is not the usual case. Such longitudinal studies also have methodologic problems, such as subject dropout for various reasons (including subsequent poor health). It was found that many of the older subjects who died during the many years of the study showed more rapid test score drops (terminal drop) in their most recent testing. This intellectual decline may reflect the impact of unexpected subclinical disease.
    4. Other approaches to measuring intelligence emphasize two components: fluid versus crystallized intelligence. Fluid intelligence reflects the degree to which the individual has developed unique qualities of thinking independent of culturally based content. Crystallized intelligence reflects the degree to which the individ-

ual has incorporated the knowledge and skills of the culture into thinking and actions.

Studies of age differences in these components show that (1) fluid intelligence decreases steadily from adolescence to at least age 60; (2) crystallized intelligence progressively increases during this time span; and (3) the magnitude of both changes is about equal, and omnibus measures (tests combining these two intelligence factors) show few age-related differences. According to other psychologists, few tests or batteries equally balance fluid and crystallized measures, so "decline" is a common finding.
5. Longitudinal studies have shown age declines only for subjects who were in their seventies or older at the start of the study.
6. Determination of true age changes in adult intellectual functioning is quite complex. Although some impairment is found, most of young adulthood, middle age, and early old age is characterized by stability or increases in intellectual performance. Decline, however, does occur relatively late in life.

C. Reaction-Time Changes (Hultsch & Deutsch, 1981, pp. 75–77; Schaie & Geiwitz, 1982, pp. 354–357)

A gradual age-related decline in reaction time occurs from the mid-twenties onward. This is found on a variety of simple performance tests, and the decrement increases with the complexity of the task and response. The overall magnitude of change is at least 20% for simple tasks and 50% or more for complex tasks. The general slowing does not appear to be primarily a function of peripheral nervous system factors (e.g., sensory acuity, speed of peripheral nerve conduction, or speed of movement once a response is initiated). Rather, it appears to reflect a basic change in the way the central nervous system processes information. The causes are unclear, but problems with brain arousal mechanisms for task preparation, decision making, and execution have been suggested. In general, reaction time does not correlate very highly with measures of intellectual ability. However, most current theorists view slowing as an integral part of emerging deficits in intellectual performance, if not capacity.

III. Sleep Changes: Polysomnography (Sleep Laboratory) Findings
(Dement, Miles, & Carskadon, 1982; Woodruff, 1985)

A. Elderly seem to spend more time in bed (TIB) (at night without attempts to sleep, unsuccessfully trying to sleep, or daytime resting or napping). The increased TIB is not due to increased total sleep time.

B. Total sleep period (TSP) is time from sleep onset to the final awakening from the main sleep period of the day. No significant change has been shown in the elderly.
C. Sleep latency (time from decision to sleep to sleep onset) is variable in the elderly, but is often greater than in younger adults.
D. Wake after sleep onset (WASO) is the time spent awake during TSP and can represent many short arousals or several long awakenings. WASO is probably the most important sleep measure regarding sleep disturbance. Many studies have found that the aged have increased amounts of WASO and increased numbers of transient arousals, three to five seconds in duration.
E. Sleep efficiency (ratio of TSP to nocturnal TIB) is frequently reduced in the elderly.
F. Sex differences in sleep pattern are observed. Elderly men seem to have objective disturbance, especially in slow wave sleep stages (SWS) and WASO, despite survey data that women have more complaints about their sleep. Whether there is a clear sex difference in objective measures of sleep in the elderly remains to be clarified.
G. Nocturnal penile tumescence (NPT) declines gradually with age during REM sleep, even though REM sleep itself, and most other REM-related variables, stay fairly constant until extreme old age.
H. Many sleep-related phenomena long considered to be normal should be regarded as important symptoms of abnormal sleep. Perhaps the most important of such phenomena is snoring.
   1. The presence of sonorous snoring may indicate some impairment of upper airway function, and in many cases, very serious impairment.
   2. There is little reliable quantitative data about the phenomenon of daytime naps in the elderly. However, studies suggest that for both sexes the total sleep time accumulated throughout an average 24-hour period (including naps) is about the same after age 60 as before age 40 (about 7.5 hours). Reports suggest that neither the amount of sleep per 24 hours nor the need for sleep decreases with age. Some investigators have shown that daytime sleepiness correlates highly with nocturnal microsleep arousals in the elderly.
I. Other Factors Affecting Sleep/Wake Function In The Elderly
   1. Prolonged bed rest (such as in bed-bound hospitalized elderly) may change the amplitudes and phases of circadian rhythms of body temperature and heart rate and may also affect the circadian sleep/wake cycle.
   2. Respiratory disturbance is defined as apnea or hypopnea during sleep; apnea is a respiratory pause of more than 10 seconds; hy-

popnea is a 50% reduction of breathing of more than 10 seconds terminating in arousal. Studies of older persons are finding a highly significant increase in respiratory disturbances in elderly compared to middle-aged subjects. Recalling that both apnea and hypopnea terminate with an arousal, data suggest that over one-third of older subjects have five or more sleep interruptions per hour. Thus, age-related respiratory impairment may account for a great deal of the sleep fragmentation in elderly subjects as reported by many investigators for both men and women. It remains to be clarified if this respiratory impairment during sleep reflects bona fide age changes or latent disease becoming manifest during sleep. Some studies suggest that in healthy elderly the rate of sleep-disordered breathing is relatively lower than that which is ascertained in community-wide studies. This suggests that the increase in sleep-disordered breathing in old age may be related to concurrent medical disease.
3. Loud snoring frequently indicates impairment of upper-airway function. The prevalence of snoring increases with age: Almost 60% of men and 45% of women in their sixties are habitual snorers. Studies measuring thoracic pressure changes in heavy snorers during sleep clearly show that airway resistance and the work of breathing are greatly increased.

J. In summary, sleep normally occupies about one-third of our daily lives during most of the adult lifespan. Sleep disturbances and sleep complaints are common in older persons. Many objective findings corroborate altered sleep function in the elderly as age-related, but some sleep disturbances (e.g., apnea) are indicative of medical or psychiatric illness.

IV. Cardiovascular Changes
(Caird & Dall, 1973; Caird, Dall, & Williams, 1985; Weisfeldt, Gerstenblith, & Lakatta, 1985)

A. Anatomy
 1. Aorta: elasticity declines with age and aortic circumference increases, primarily due to changes in the aortic media; there is a resultant increase in pulse amplitude and systolic BP (but little change in diastolic BP).
 2. Heart valves: several age-related changes occur in the valve cusps and rings and in the "fibrous skeleton" of the heart.
    a. Aortic valve: there is steady age-related progression of decreased nuclei in the fibrous stroma of the valve, an accumulation of lipid, degeneration of collagen and elastosis, and calcifi-

cation in the valve fibrosa; increased valve stiffness probably causes the common systolic murmur of the elderly, and the changes probably predispose to calcific aortic sclerosis without commisural fusion; extension of the calcific process into the interventricular septum may be a cause of bundle branch block.
  b. Mitral valve: similar to aortic valve changes but less severe for any given age; also, the close relation of the main bundle of His to the mitral ring may result in varying degrees of heart block.
  c. Tricuspid and pulmonary valves: essentially similar changes but of lesser magnitude and frequency than in the aortic and mitral valves.
 3. Myocardium: "brown atrophy" (a decrease in heart weight plus an accumulation of lipofuscin in the myocardial fibers) occurs; other age-related changes (fibrotic lesions and senile amyloidosis) may represent disease rather than true age changes; mild left ventricular wall hypertrophy partly reflecting increased aortic input impedence manifests as an increase in systolic B.P.
B. Function
 1. Cardiac output: generally not affected by age at rest, but dynamic exercise studies have shown a decrease either in cardiac output, heart rate, or ejection fraction under the stress of exercise.
 2. Heart rate: resting heart rate not notably affected by age; an age-associated decrease in heart rate response under exercise stress workload (compensated for by an age-associated increase in stroke volume via heightened use of Frank-Starling mechanism since cardiac output is maintained).
C. Clinical Importance: The above changes make it clinically important to be vigilant regarding cardiovascular side effects when antidepressants or neuroleptics are prescribed. The interaction between these age-related changes and psychiatric medications may convert potential to actual clinically significant cardiovascular dysfunction. This is especially true because cardiovascular disease is especially prevalent in the elderly.

V. Pulmonary Changes
(Freeman, 1985; Culver & Butler, 1985)

A. Anatomic and Functional Changes
 1. Lung volumes: progressive fall in vital capacity (VC) and in forced expiratory volume in one second (FEV:1); residual volume

(RV) increases with age and accounts for an increasing proportion of the total lung capacity (TLC).
2. Ventilatory distribution: increased ventilation-perfusion mismatch due to alveolar septal loss, vacuolar, and other changes.
3. Diffusing capacity: significantly decreases with age.
4. Blood gas changes: the alveolar-arterial oxygen difference increases with age due mainly to a progressive fall in arterial oxygen pressure; the arterial carbon dioxide pressure is unchanged with aging.
5. Respiratory disturbances during sleep (see section III on "Sleep Changes"). These disturbances are the most clinically relevant pulmonary changes for the practicing psychiatrist.

VI. Endocrine Changes

A. Hypothalamic-Neurohypophyseal-Renal Axis (Halderman, 1982): Antidiuretic hormone (arginine vasopressin, AVP) is secreted by the posterior pituitary and is under two control systems: (1) hypothalamic osmoreceptors and (2) noncentral neurogenic controls. The kidney retains nearly normal responsiveness to AVP with aging. The aging kidney maintains relatively normal urine concentration but fails to maximally concentrate or dilute when water is withheld or provided in excess. The failure to maximally concentrate is due to altered driving forces for water movement (renal osmotic gradients) and not caused by renal unresponsiveness to AVP. One clinical consequence is that older depressives with reduced appetite and decreased fluid intake may lose weight rather rapidly until the depression is adequately treated.
B. Hypothalamic-Pituitary-Adrenal Axis (Wolfsen, 1982; Blichert-Toft, 1978)
  1. Hypothalamus secretes corticotrophin releasing hormone (CRH) into the hypophyseal-portal blood and stimulates pituitary ACTH secretion. CRH release is regulated by higher brain centers, including the limbic system, and follows a circadian rhythm in which ACTH and cortisol have frequent secretory bursts during the early morning hours.
  2. With Aging
    a. Glucocorticoid production—the circadian rhythm of cortisol—remains intact: plasma total and unbound corticosteroid responses following ACTH stimulation are unaltered in advanced age.
    b. Adrenal androgens show an age-related reduction to about 50% of normal in people over age 60.

c. Aldosterone: secretion rate is lowered in healthy, elderly persons. Possible age changes in renin levels and development of nephrosclerosis may be contributing factors.
   d. Adrenal medullary function: slight age-related decreases in epinephrine and norepinephrine excretion; dopamine excretion is somewhat raised.
   e. Dexamethasone suppression test (DST): it is unsettled whether or not advancing age affects the prevalence of abnormal DST results in normal older persons. Data suggest that advanced age affects higher post-DST cortisol levels in patients with depression or dementia (Georgotas et al., 1986; Greenwald et al., 1986).
C. Hypothalamic-Anterior Pituitary-Thyroid Axis (Melmed & Hershman, 1982)
   1. TRH stimulates the release of TSH. Circulating thyroid hormones inhibit TSH release and the responsivity of the pituitary to the stimulatory effect of TRH.
   2. The upper normal limits of free serum T3 and T4 are probably unchanged with age. Old age is accompanied by lower T3 levels, with relatively normal or slightly decreased T4 levels.
   3. Thyrotropin (TSH) serum levels are generally normal; small elevations probably represent primary hypothyroidism rather than "normal" levels. The feedback response of circulating thyroid hormones at the pituitary level is also intact in the elderly.
D. Age-Related Changes in Carbohydrate Metabolism (Davidson, 1982)
   1. A progressive age-related decline in glucose tolerance has been demonstrated in many studies. Most studies using an oral glucose tolerance test (OGTT) find an age-related decline in glucose tolerance. The magnitude of change is approximately 9.5 mg % per decade for one-hour values and about 5.3 mg % per decade for two-hour values. Simpler postprandial glucose tests within one to two hours of eating rise some 4 mg % per decade (Davidson, 1982, pp. 232-233). There are significant anatomic changes in the pancreas with aging, such as fatty infiltration and atrophy of islet cells.
   2. Insulin secretion: there seems to be no age-related impairment in the amount of pancreatic insulin available for secretion, the half-life and metabolic clearance rate of insulin, or fasting insulin concentrations. The relationship between aging and insulin secretion after various stimuli (oral and intravenous) is not yet clear; some studies show no change and others show delayed, increased, or decreased insulin response.

3. Insulin action: a number of studies suggest that older subjects have impaired insulin action and that the peripheral tissues (muscle and fat) are the site of insulin antagonism in aging.
4. Summary: up to 50% of patients over age 60 have abnormal glucose tolerance tests with normal FBS levels. The underlying causes of this change are not clearly understood.

VII. Changes in Female and Male Reproductive Function (See Chapter 3, this volume, on sexuality in the elderly)

VIII. Gastrointestinal Changes (Texter, 1983; Bhanthumnavin & Schuster, 1977)

A. Esophagus: tendency toward decreased motility and increased failures of lower esophageal sphincter to relax after swallowing, with delay in esophageal emptying time in the elderly.
B. Stomach: hyposecretion of acid, intrinsic factors, and pepsin; increased incidence of atrophic gastritis; diminished absorption of iron and vitamin B12 as a result of these physiological changes.
C. Small intestine: in general, there is little or no evidence that diminished absorption of nutrients occurs in normal elderly persons; there is little evidence of major difference in drug absorption in healthy older subjects (Texter, 1983, p. 48). However, studies have shown a decrease of iron and calcium absorption with aging.
D. Colon: increasing occurrence with age of constipation and diverticulosis.
E. Liver: gradual age-related reduction in hepatic blood flow; hepatocyte loss with a decreased serum albumin; likely reduction in drug metabolizing system in the microsomes, with impairment of metabolism of some (but not all) drugs. Reduction of serum albumin can lead to an increase of unbound active drug. The combination of reduced metabolism of drugs and increase in the unbound fraction can lead to higher blood levels of active drug and hence an increased risk of side effects.
F. Gall bladder: no clear age-related changes.
G. In summary, gastrointestinal disease and symptoms are prevalent in the elderly. They are usually not age-related changes and must be seriously evaluated as indicators of physical or psychiatric illness. Some age-related changes, such as those in the liver, can have important implications in the use of psychotropic medications.

IX. Renal Changes
(Rowe, Andres, Tobin, Norris, & Shock, 1976; Foster & Rosenthal, 1980)

A progressive age-related decrease in renal clearance because of progressive loss of nephroma occurs from age 30 onward. The magnitude of this change is at least a 30% decrease from ages 30 to 80 and may accelerate after age 65. The impairment does not usually manifest itself in elevations of blood urea nitrogen (BUN) or creatinine levels. It is easily measured by a 24-hour creatinine clearance study. This decline has important implications for drug metabolism in general, and particularly for the safe use of lithium salts in the elderly. It is an important factor in the general need for lower dosage of psychotropic drugs in the elderly.

X. Immunologic Changes
(Weksler, 1982, 1983; Adler & Nagel, 1985; Fox, 1985).

A. Involution of thymus gland: a universal 90% to 95% reduction of maximal mass from sexual maturity to ages 45–50 occurs; this involution during the first half of life may explain the altered form and function of the immune system seen during the second half of life.
B. Lymphocytes
   1. Total number of lymphocytes, including T- or B-lymphocytes in the blood, does not change with age; however,
   2. Significant redistribution of lymphoid compartments occurs with aging (e.g., decrease in germinal centers in lymph nodes and an increase in plasma cells and lymphocytes in the bone marrow).
   3. Proportions of T-lymphocyte subpopulations change in peripheral blood with aging (e.g., increase in immature T-lymphocytes, decrease in helper T-cells, and an increase in T-suppressors).
   4. With aging, there is increased susceptibility to damage induced by ionizing radiation, ultraviolet light, and mutagenic drugs.
C. Humoral Immunity
   1. There is little change in total serum immunoglobulin concentration; macrophage function appears unchanged; however,
   2. Distribution of immunoglobin class changes with age (Ig M decreases; Ig A and Ig G increases).
   3. Autoantibodies and monoclonal immunoglobulins increase with aging.
   4. Response to foreign antigens decreases with age.
   5. Thus, the humoral response is often impaired in older persons;

this is predominantly due to a decrease in helper T-cell activity, although increased suppressor activity and deficits in B-lymphocyte function may also play a role.
D. Cell-Mediated Immunity
   1. Cell-mediated immunity (e.g., delayed hypersensitivity and graft rejection) depends on the functional integrity of thymic-dependent lymphocytes.
   2. Some elderly may have less vigorous or absent delayed hypersensitivity reactions to common skin-testing antigen, though many healthy older adults have normal responses.
   3. *In vitro* tests of lymphocytes from old persons show impaired proliferative response to T-lymphocyte mitogens. This deficit appears to be due to decreased numbers of mitogen-responsive T-lymphocytes, reflecting impaired proliferative capacity of those mitogen-responsive cells in culture.
   4. Thus, cell-mediated immunity is impaired in many older humans. The anergy probably has clinical consequences regarding longevity and may also contribute to the reactivation of such diseases as tuberculosis and varicella zoster (shingles) (Fox, 1985, p. 89).
E. In summary, the increased susceptibility of the elderly to infections, neoplastic disease, and perhaps vascular damage may be a consequence of immune senescence. The contribution of autoantibodies to the pathobiology of aging is less certain.
F. Possible relevance to psychiatric illness: various studies have suggested short-term (about 6 months) altered immune function in bereavement, depression, and schizophrenia as well as other stress states (see Udelman & Udelman, 1983; Schindler, 1985; Stein, 1986). These studies have not thus far suggested a more direct link between normal aging, immune senescence, and psychiatric illness. However, it is possible that further work could generate new hypotheses concerning interactions among these axes.

REFERENCES

Adler, W. H., & Nagel, J. F. (1985). Clinical immunology. In R. Andres, E. L. Bierman, & W. R. Hazzard (Eds.), *Principles of geriatric medicine* (pp. 413–423). New York: McGraw-Hill.

Blichert-Toft, M. (1978). The adrenal glands in old age. In R. B. Greenblatt (Ed.), *Geriatric endocrinology* (pp. 81–102). New York: Raven Press.

Caird, F. I., & Dall, J. L. C. (1973). The cardiovascular system. In J. C. Brocklehurst (Ed.), *Textbook of geriatric medicine and gerontology* (pp. 122–160). London: Churchill Livingstone.

Caird, F. I., Dall, J. L. C., & Williams, B. O. (1985). The cardiovascular system. In J. C. Brocklehurst (Ed.), *Textbook of geriatric medicine and gerontology* (3rd ed.) (pp. 230-267). New York: Churchill Livingstone.

Corso, J. (1977). Auditory perception and communication. In J. E. Birren & K. W. Schaie (Eds.), *Handbook of the psychology of aging* (pp. 535-561). New York: Van Nostrand Reinhold.

Culver, B. H., & Butler, J. (1985). Alterations in pulmonary function. In R. Andres, E. L. Bierman, & W. R. Hazzard (Eds.), *Principles of geriatric medicine* (pp. 280-287). New York: McGraw-Hill.

Davidson, J. M. (1985). Sexuality and aging. In R. Andres, E. L. Bierman, & W. R. Hazzard (Eds.), *Principles of geriatric medicine* (pp. 154-161). New York: McGraw-Hill.

Davidson, M. B. (1982). The effect of aging on carbohydrate metabolism: A comprehensive review and a practical approach to the clinical problem. In S. G. Korenman (Ed.), *Endocrine aspects of aging* (pp. 231-267). New York: Elsevier Biomedical.

Dement, W. C., Miles, L. E., & Carskadon, M. A. (1982). "White paper" on sleep and aging. *Journal of the American Geriatrics Society, 30,* 25-50.

Fisch, L. (1985). Special senses: The aging auditory system. In J. C. Brocklehurst (Ed.), *Textbook of geriatric medicine and gerontology* (pp. 484-499). New York: Churchill Livingstone.

Foster, J. R., & Rosenthal, J. S. (1980). Lithium treatment of the elderly. In F. W. Johnson (Ed.), *Handbook of lithium therapy* (pp. 414-420). Baltimore: United Park Press.

Fox, R. A. (1985). Immunology of aging. In J. C. Brocklehurst (Ed.), *Textbook of geriatric medicine and gerontology* (3rd ed.) (pp. 82-104). New York: Churchill Livingstone.

Fozard, J. L., Wolf, E., Bell, B., McFarland, R. A., & Podolsky, S. (1977). Visual perception and communication. In J. E. Birren & K. W. Schaie (Eds.), *Handbook of the psychology of aging* (pp. 497-534). New York: Van Nostrand Reinhold.

Freeman, E. (1985). The respiratory system. In J. C. Brocklehurst (Ed.), *Textbook of geriatric medicine and gerontology* (pp. 731-757). New York: Churchill Livingstone.

Georgotas, A., McCue, R. E., Kim, O. M., Hapsworth, W. E., Reisberg, B., Stoll, P. M., Sinaiko, E., Fanelli, C., & Stokes, P. E. (1986). Dexamethasone suppression in dementia, depression and normal aging. *American Journal of Psychiatry, 143,* 452-456.

Greenwald, B. S., Mathe, A. A., Mohs, R. C., Levy, M. I., Johns, C. A., & Davis, K. L. (1986). Cortisol and Alzheimer's disease, II. Dexamethasone suppression, dementia severity, and affective symptoms. *American Journal of Psychiatry, 143,* 442-446.

Halderman, J. H. (1982). The impact of normal aging on the hypothalamic-neurohypophyseal-renal axis. In S. G. Korenman (Ed.), *Endocrine aspects of aging* (pp. 9-32). New York: Elsevier Biomedical.

Hultsch, D. F., & Deutsch, F. (1981). *Adult development and aging.* New York: McGraw-Hill.

Huyck, M. H., & Hoyer, W. J. (1982). *Adult development and aging.* Belmont, CA: Wadsworth.

Judd, H. L., & Korenman, S. G. (1982). Effects of aging on reproductive function in women. In S. G. Korenman (Ed.), *Endocrine aspects of aging* (pp. 163-230). New York: Elsevier Biomedical.

Kaplan, H. S. (1974). *The new sex therapy.* New York: Brunner/Mazel.

Kline, D. W., & Schieber, F. (1985). Vision and aging. In J. E. Birren & K. W. Schaie (Eds.), *Handbook of the psychology of aging* (pp. 296-331). New York: Van Nostrand Reinhold.

Masters, W. H., & Johnson, V. E. (1970). *Human sexual inadequacy.* Boston: Little, Brown.

Melmed, S., & Hershman, J. M. (1982). The thyroid and aging. In S. G. Korenman (Ed.), *Endocrine aspects of aging* (pp. 33-53). New York: Elsevier Biomedical.

Olsho, L. W., Harkins, S. W., & Lenhardt, M. L. (1985). Aging and the auditory system. In J. E. Birren & K. W. Schaie (Eds.), *Handbook of the psychology of aging* (pp. 332-377). New York: Van Nostrand Reinhold.

Rowe, J. W., Andres, R., Tobin, J. D., Norris, A. M., & Shock, N. W. (1976). The effect of age on creative clearance in men: A cross-sectional and longitudinal study. *Journal of Gerontology, 31,* 155-163.

Schaie, K. W., & Geiwitz, J. (1982). *Adult development and aging.* Boston: Little, Brown.

Schindler, B. A. (1985). Stress, affective disorders and immune function. *Medical Clinics of North America, 69*(3), 585-597.

Stein, M. (1986). A reconsideration of specificity in psychosomatic medicine: From olfaction to the lymphocyte. *Psychosomatic Medicine, 48,* 3-22.

Texter, E. C. (Ed.). (1983). *The aging gut.* New York: Masson Publishing USA.

Udelman, H. D., & Udelman, D. L. (1983). Current explorations in psychoimmunology. *American Journal of Psychotherapy, 37*(2), 210-221.

Weisfeldt, M. L., Gerstenblith, G., & Lakatta, E. G. (1985). Alterations in circulatory function. In R. Andres, E. L. Bierman, & W. R. Hazzard (Eds.), *Principles of geriatric medicine* (pp. 248-279). New York: McGraw-Hill.

Weksler, M. E. (1982). Age-associated changes in the immune response. *Journal of the American Geriatrics Society, 30,* 718-723.

Weksler, M. E. (1983). Senescence of the immune system. *Medical Clinics of North America, 67*(2), 263-272.

Wolfsen, A. R. (1982). Aging and the adrenals. In S. G. Korenman (Ed.), *Endocrine aspects of aging* (pp. 55-80). New York: Elsevier Biomedical.

Woodruff, D. S. (1985). Arousal, sleep, and aging. In J. E. Birren & K. W. Schaie (Eds.), *Handbook of the psychology of aging* (pp. 261-295). New York: Van Nostrand Reinhold.

3
Sexuality and Sexual Dysfunction in the Elderly

Eugene M. Dagon

I. Sexuality in Normal Aging and Disease

Ageism denotes the collection of negative societal attitudes toward the elderly. Ageist attitudes on the part of clinicians are prime determinants in limiting care of the elderly. Although there have been many advances in the diagnosis and treatment of sexual dysfunctions, actual practice often proceeds from deficient medical school curricula, anecdotal knowledge, and ageist attitudes of diagnostic and therapeutic nihilism.

Physicians, as part of an often ageist and sexist society, frequently do not inquire into the sexual histories and practices of their aging patients. Burnap and Golden (1967) have noted that two-thirds of physicians who inquire into sexual practices of their patients note significant dysfunctions in at least half of them, whereas those physicians who do not routinely inquire about sexual practices estimate that less than 10% of their patients have sexual problems.

Sexual functioning serves as a natural buffer against many of the stresses and losses accompanying aging. Unfortunately, many of the medications and chronic illnesses accompanying aging deprive elderly patients prematurely and inappropriately of sexual functioning.

The purpose of this chapter is to review the normal sexual changes of aging and thus allow the physician to recognize and deal more effectively with the myths, maladies, and medications that lead to sexual dysfunction. The physician's standard of practice should be to preserve, restore, and promote sensuality and sexuality among his or her aging patients.

The following are some of the more common myths that affect sexuality in later life.

A. Chronology myth (Butler & Lewis, 1976). This myth assumes that sexuality automatically diminishes with advancing age until one becomes old and asexual. Some studies (Bengtson, Cuellar, & Ragan, 1977) have shown that large numbers of individuals in ethnic subgroups hold similar arbitrary views and define old age as a certain chronological time of life or decade, for example, after age 50 among Chicanos, after age 60 among blacks, after age 70 among Causcasians. While there is some sexual decline with aging, there are a number of intervening variables—such as disease, presence of a partner, and attitudes and adaptation to aging—that have more to do with sexual functioning than chronological aging per se. Pfeiffer (1974), in reviewing the Duke longitudinal aging studies, offered the following facts:

- at age 63, about 70% of men were still sexually active
- at age 78, 25% of men were sexually active
- for men, the married state was not a necessary factor for continued coital activity
- for women, the availability of a socially sanctioned mate was a factor for continued coital activity

B. Tranquility myth (Butler & Lewis, 1976). This refers to the assumed blissful asexual golden age when a person is free from sexual concerns and passions. Pfeiffer (1974) noted that there was no decade this side of a hundred in which there were not some age cohorts who were coitally active.

C. Guilt and shame myth (Glover, 1978). This derives from the attitude during the Victorian era, when sex was considered "dirty," an attitude frequently stated as "nice girls don't" or "women have duties to submit to the pleasure of men, but do not take pleasure in such things themselves."

D. Second-class sexual myth (Dagon, 1983). This refers to the close association of sexual identity with personal identity and socioeconomic status. Many elderly people experience socioeconomic decline after retirement. Although for most elderly the decade from age 65 to age 75 is a healthy one, some experience major health problems that strain their decreased financial resources. Some become frail and/or medically indigent. Although Medicare (Title 18) insurance is an entitlement, many elderly view public funding as denoting second-class status. This view is particularly reinforced by the limited reimbursement for Medicaid (Title 19) patients. Many clinicians refuse or limit their services to Title 18 and Title 19 patients. These patients may then be limited to public-sector health services. In the public sector, sexual problems or needs are often regarded as of secondary or limited importance and therefore do not warrant the clinician's concern.

E. Frugality myth (Dagon, 1983). This refers to the cultural idea that sexuality is of limited quantity and needs to be saved. However, sexual behavior is learned behavior and performance is enhanced with practice and positive reinforcement. Unless there is educational exposure to refute this myth, disuse atrophy may lead to sexual dysfunction.

F. Stereotypic role myth. Sometimes referred to as the sleeping-beauty-and-prince-charming myth, this assumption is that women are neither initiators of sex nor responsible for their own sexuality (i.e., they must wait passively for the male to initiate sex by awakening the princess with a kiss). Many older men experience anxiety about the normal changes of aging, such as the need for greater stimulation to achieve an erection, but become uncomfortable with a woman who initiates sex. Couples who do not have permission, or information, to change cultural stereotypic behaviors often experience sexual dysfunction with aging.

G. Ignorance is bliss myth. This assumes that the elderly are not interested in sexual functioning and that the health practitioner need not inquire into an area in which he or she has received limited medical school training. If the elderly patient were truly interested in his or her sexual problem, he or she would ask. Masters and Johnson (1970) have noted that fully 50% of couples experience sexual dysfunction at some time during their lives. Everyone could therefore benefit from accurate sexual information.

H. Menopause myth. This refers to the assumption that menopause marks the end of sexual functioning. In reality, reproductive capacity is only a portion of the individual's sexual capacity throughout the life cycle.

I. Masturbation myth. This refers to the Victorian attitude that masturbation is a symptom of a "weak mind" and can cause mental illness. Although this myth has no scientific basis, it is nonetheless surprising to find elderly people who harbor this attitude, which they may have learned in childhood. Studies have noted that 90% of males and 50% females in the 1940s and 1950s masturbated (Kinsey, 1948, 1953). The sexual revolution of women in the past few decades has effected female masturbatory activity approximating the male rates.

J. Stroke and heart attack myths (Hellerstein, 1970; Ueno, 1963). This refers to the common belief that sexual functioning is so physically demanding that coitus may precipitate a heart attack, stroke, or even death. This myth supports the idea that if one's spouse has cardiovascular disease, sexual abstinence should be practiced to lessen these dangers. The occurrence of death during coitus is quite rare; however, the fantasy of death during coitus often causes many couples to abandon sexual activity. Studies have shown that the physical demands of coitus with a familiar partner (e.g., a spouse) are approximately the same as those of mild exercise activities that the patient is capable of performing.
K. Dirty old man myth. This refers in part to the double standard that old men have sex on their mind but not old women. Many postmenopausal women report increased sexual desire after menopause. Studies suggest that women are capable of orgasm well into advanced old age. In similar age cohorts, sexual potency in men declines slowly. Sensuality has been shown to be important to both sexes as they age, although the biological capability for sex may be greater for the woman than for the man. It is time to recognize that the cultural myth regarding the "dirty old man" is inaccurate, and that sexual initiative may reside more with "dirty old women," while the preservation and promotion of sensuality and sexuality in the elderly should be the standard for both sexes.
L. Homosexual myth. This assumes that most homosexuals are mentally disturbed and do not age as well as their heterosexual age cohorts. The referendum in psychiatry that changed the categorization of homosexuality from the realm of psychopathology to that of sexual preference is relatively recent. The evidence regarding homosexuals adapting to the aging process is still not clear. Some authors (Kelly, 1977; Kimmel, 1978) claim that being homosexual allows men sex-role flexibility, thus facilitating adaptation to aging, and that the male homosexual subculture encourages self-interest and narcissism, which may aid adaptation to some of the losses of aging. Some authors (Hart et al., 1978) claim that the lesbian subculture is more supportive of age-related changes in aging partners.
M. Terminal asexual myth (Jaffe, 1977). This refers to the belief that the dying patient is devoid of sexuality. Confronting death means coming to grips with the existential state of nonbeing. Some thanatologists note that death anxiety is diminished with the ability of the dying to savor the present moment. Sunrises, the textures and colors of nature, sensuality, touch, holding and being held by a loved sexual intimate, whether it is with or without coital activity, is important to the dying patient.

N. Procreation, not recreation, myth (Dagon, 1983). This refers to the belief, fostered by some religious groups, that coital activity is only for procreation. While procreation is a proper object of coital activity, the exclusive focus on it fails to recognize the narrow range of reproductive maturity in comparison to sexual capacity throughout the life cycle and the role of sexual relations in the formation of stable pair-bonding and intimacy.
O. Asexual chronic disease myth (Gurian, 1986). This refers to the belief that all elderly with chronic diseases are too ill to care about sex. Some physicians prescribe sexual abstinence for a number of acute illnesses, such as myocardial infarcts, urinary tract infections, low back pain, and some emotional disorders. However, sexual needs may become more prominent with improvement or recovery from a chronic illness. It is noteworthy that 50% of people over the age of 60, and 80% over the age of 70, have chronic health problems and that their sexual concerns need the attention and expertise of their physician. Countertransference in the clinician often limits care of sexual dysfunctions that are potentially reversible in chronic disease.

II. Normal Sexual Response Cycle Associated with Normal Aging
(Pfeiffer, 1974; Verwoerdt, 1969; Masters & Johnson, 1966)

A. Major changes commonly occur in the sexual response patterns of the aging male.
  1. Longer time period during the excitement phase to achieve full erection; males need greater use of fantasy, foreplay, and stimulation.
  2. More difficulty than young men in maintaining a full erection.
  3. Lengthening of the plateau phase so that there is a better opportunity for ejaculatory control.
  4. A lessening of desire for orgasm.
  5. Decrease in the force and amount of the ejaculate.
B. Major changes also commonly occur in the sexual response patterns of the aging female.
  1. As with males, an increase in the excitatory threshold so that more time is required to obtain lubrication.
  2. With thinning of the vaginal mucosa postmenopausally, there is decreased lubrication.
  3. Increased desire for sexual activity in late middle-age, with a gradual decline of sexual interest in old age.
  4. The continued ability to have orgasms as long as physically healthy.

C. Summary of Normal Sexual Responses
   1. The four stages described by Masters and Johnson (1966, 1970) are (1) excitement, (2) plateau, (3) orgasm, and (4) resolution.
   2. The triphasic stages described by Kaplan (1971) are (1) desire, (2) excitement, and (3) orgasm.

III. Components of Sexual Dysfunction (Kaplan, 1974)

A. From the Individual Viewpoint—Immediate Causes
   1. Individual sexual behavior—failure to engage in effective sexual behavior, sexual function is constricted, mechanical and orgasm-oriented because of misinformation and ignorance.
   2. Sexual Anxiety
      a. Fear of failure—anticipatory anxiety-failure cycle.
      b. Demand for performance.
      c. Excessive need to please partner.
   3. Perceptual and Intellectual Defenses Against Erotic Feelings
      a. spectator role.
      b. denial.
   4. Communication Failures
B. From the Systems Viewpoint: Current factors such as stress, disease, and life-cycle stages, coupled with historical factors, past learning, and cultural and religious upbringing, all play a role in the aged person's sexual functioning. This may be visualized as in Figure 3.1.

   At any point in time, a cross-section of the life-cycle cylinder may be conceptualized as in Figure 3.2.

   These biopsychosocial factors may be further developed into the factors listed in Table 3.1.

IV. Physical Illnesses Commonly Affecting Sexual Function (Griffith & Trieschmann, 1983; Renshaw, 1985; Wise, 1978, 1983)

A. Introduction
   1. Approximately 90% of sexual dysfunctions secondary to physical illness are functional in origin (Kaplan, 1974). However, with aging, organic causes play an increasing role in sexual dysfunction.
   2. The diseases that have the greatest effect on sexual functioning are primarily diseases of the genitourinary system and, secondarily, diseases of secondary sexual organs.

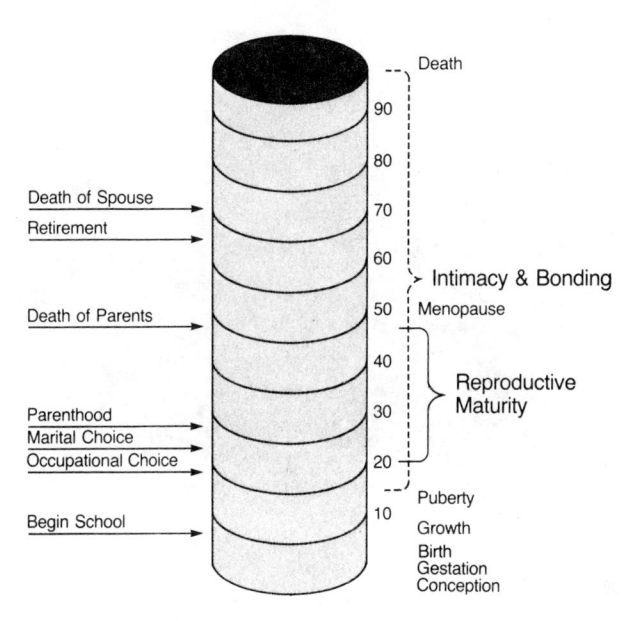

Sexuality and Sexual Dysfunction in the Elderly   47

FIGURE 3.1 Life-span sexual development by decades with approximate impact of life stress units.

Source: Dagon, 1983. Reprinted by permission of Plenum Publishing Corp.

TABLE 3.1 Biopsychosocial Parameters of Function

Biodynamic factors	Psychodynamic factors	Sociocultural dynamic factors
Anatomic and physiologic changes of aging	Intrapsychic and interpersonal changes accompanying aging	Environmental changes
Genetic	Personality type	Socioeconomic status: income, poverty, housing
Environmental	Intelligence, creative abilities	Ethnic and racial background
Surgical	Defenses and coping styles	Cultural values
Traumatic	Object losses, e.g., death of spouse, divorce, marital separation, status, role, income	Family support systems
Infectious		Community networks
Toxic		Shame-vs.-guilt cultures
Metabolic	Dyadic relations: marital, parent–child	Culture age-graded for male and female roles
Endocrine	Family support system	

Source: Dagon, 1983. Reprinted by permission of Plenum Publishing Corp.

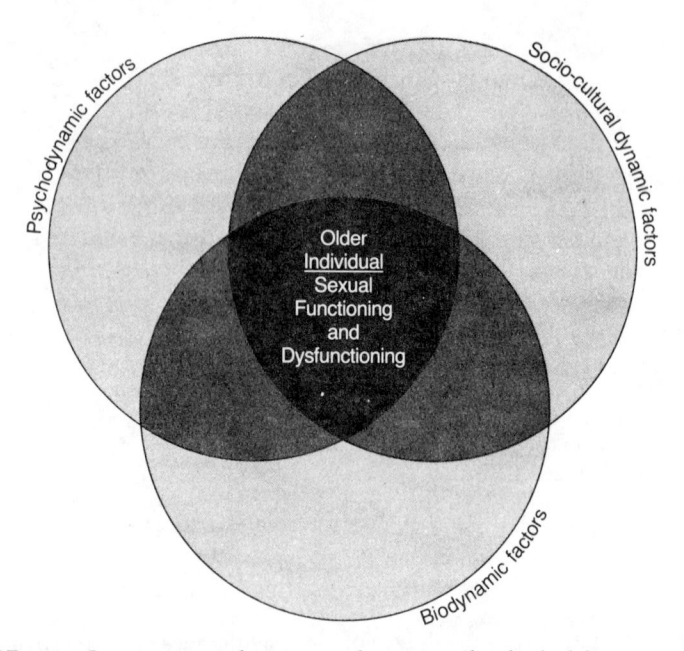

FIGURE 3.2 Cross-sectional moment along an individual's life span. The area of sexual functioning has been separated into biopsychosociocultural components.

Source: Dagon, 1983. Reprinted by permission of Plenum Publishing Corp.

    3. Other common systemic diseases affecting sexual fuctioning include cardiovascular, respiratory, and endocrine ailments.
    4. Patients are concerned about sexual functioning, even when acutely ill, but often fail to discuss sexual issues with their physician unless the physician specifically inquires.
B. Primary Diseases of the Genitourinary Tract
    1. Prostate Disease (Ellis & Grayhack, 1963; Finkle & Prian, 1966; Finkle, 1975, 1978; Furlow, 1980; Herr, 1979; Jonas, 1983; Madorsky, Drylie, & Finlayson, 1976; Walsh & Mostwin, 1984)
        a. Over 50% of older men develop benign prostatic hypertrophy (BPH).
        b. Many who have transurethral resection of the prostate (TURP) will develop impotence for psychological, not physiological, reasons.
        c. Retrograde ejaculation may occur post-TURP, with semen being deposited in the urinary bladder, causing infertility but not impotence.

d. Cancer surgery with perineal or suprapubic approaches can disrupt parasympathetic fibers from S_2, S_3, and S_4 and may cause erectile failures with a physiological basis. The incidence of ejaculation difficulties with or without concomitant erectile failure has been 78% following retropubic, and 100% following perineal, prostatectomy. Walsh and Mostwin (1984) have reported modified retropubic prostatectomy techniques that appear to preserve potency in two-thirds of the patients.
e. Sexual functioning may be preserved by treating cancer with iodine 125 or gold 198 implants. After iodine treatment, erectile difficulties occurred in 13% and retrograde ejaculation occurred in approximately 28% of patients.
f. Erectile dysfunction generally has been reported by 20% to 40% of patients irradiated for cancer of the prostate.
g. Two major types of penile prostheses are available for organically caused impotence: semi-rigid rod (Small-Carrion) and inflatable hydraulic (Scott-Bradley).

2. Menopause (Carr & MacDonald, 1985; Glowacki, 1978; Gordan & Vaughan, 1977; Ziel & Finkle, 1975)
   a. Median age for cessation of menstrual bleeding (female climacteric) is 50–51 years.
   b. Principal endocrine changes that characterize the climacteric are due primarily to decreased cyclic ovarian estrogen secretion.
   c. Menopausal syndrome includes hot flashes (vasomotor instability), dryness and atrophy of urogenital epithelium and vagina, osteoporosis, and psychological symptoms (insomnia, irritability, and rapid mood swings).
   d. In many studies, postmenopausal women noted no major discontinuity in life and, except for the underlying biological changes, they had a relative degree of control over their menopausal symptoms.
   e. Low-dose estrogen is effective for treatment of hot flashes and urogenital atrophy.
   f. Urogenital atrophy is associated with dyspareunia, vaginismus, and decreased sexual desire.
   g. Estrogen is beneficial for preventing symptoms of osteoporosis in young oophorectomized women. If given in low doses three years prior to menopause, estrogen may prevent fractures in older women.
   h. After three years of estrogen deficiency, bone changes from estrogen deficiency are irreversible.

i. The risk of endometrial cancer is 5 to 14 times higher in women treated with estrogens compared with untreated controls.
j. All women on estrogen therapy should be evaluated semiannually for increased blood pressure, breast masses, and endometrial hyperplasia.

3. Hysterectomy (Jackson, 1979; Nadelson, 1977)
   a. Hysterectomy is the most commonly performed major surgery in the United States.
   b. Hysterectomy does not produce significant psychopathology in the majority of women, but it is associated with a grief reaction associated with the psychological significance of the uterus as a symbol of femininity and generativity. A brief period of mourning with gender reintegration is usual.
   c. The most frequent psychopathologic reaction to hysterectomy is depression.
   d. Factors associated with higher risk of psychopathology following hysterectomy include poor gender identity, previous and adverse reactions to stress, previous depression/anxiety, family history of depression, history of multiple somatic complaints, younger age, anxiety that surgery will cause diminished sexual capacity, marital instability and perceived rejection by spouse, limited avocational interests to serve as alternative means of satisfaction, and religious or ethnocultural negative attitudes regarding hysterectomy.
   e. Dyspareunia may be associated with decreased lubrication or narrowing and stenosis of the vagina, especially in patients who have had substantial posterior colpoperineorrhapies.
   f. Counseling strategies to prevent sexual dysfunction following hysterectomy may focus on physical and psychological goals.
      (1) Physical Goals
         (a) Sexual abstinence until six-weeks postoperative visit, when patient is checked for adhesions and quality of healing.
         (b) Resuming of sexual activity after six-weeks visit.
         (c) Avoidance of deep penetration that is uncomfortable.
         (d) Increased time of foreplay to assure maximal lubrication and/or utilization of a lubricant (e.g., K-Y jelly).
      (2) Psychological Goals
         (a) Education that hysterectomy does not adversely affect a woman's femininity or sexual desire and responsiveness (many women report increased sexual responsiveness when relieved of fears of pregnancy).

(b) Allowing time to complete a period of mourning and gender reintegration.
(c) Exploring and encouraging communication between spouses that reaffirms mutual desirability.
(d) Identifying early unresolved grief, marital dysfunction, or high-risk indicators that would require psychiatric referral and/or counseling.
4. Vaginismus (McGuire, Guzinski, & Holmes, 1980; Tollison & Adam, 1979)
   a. Recurrent and persistent involuntary spasm of the musculature (bulbocavernous and levator muscles) of the outer one-third of the vagina that interferes with coitus.
   b. With vaginismus, repeated attempts at intercourse lead to dyspareunia, intense anxiety, and phobic avoidance behavior.
   c. Physical factors that produce painful intercourse and may lead to vaginismus as an acquired response include endometriosis, relaxation of the supporting uterine ligaments, senile atrophy of the vagina with stenosis, pelvic inflammatory disease, pelvic tumors, and urethral caruncles.
   d. Psychodynamic factors contributing to vaginismus include a defense against overt or psychological trauma and guilt; traumatic psychological factors may include rape, painful loss of virginity, dyspareunia, or intense guilt reactions resulting from strict religious rearing, fear of pregnancy, or reaction to repeated erectile failures or premature ejaculations.
   e. Treatment strategies include:
      (1) Psychoanalytic—bring into consciousness and resolve repressed guilt or anger toward spouse or men.
      (2) Medical or surgical—perineotomy to enlarge vaginal orifice and/or pharmacological therapy with anxiolytics and smooth muscle relaxants.
      (3) Behavior therapy.
         (a) Systematic desensitization of anxiety and reduction of phobic elements.
         b) *In vivo* extinction of the spastic vaginal response.
C. Diseases of Secondary Sexual Organs
   1. Mastectomy (Abt, McGurrin, & Heintz, 1978; Asken, 1975; Ervin, 1973; Frank, 1978; Witkin, 1975)
      a. Visible mutilation may have more traumatic effects than nonvisible loss of the uterus.
      b. Female issues include those of self-image and the negative response of the man; male issues relate to his nonverbal communication of rejection.

c. Return to sexual functioning is enhanced by early inclusion of the husband and significant others in rehabilitation (e.g., dressing changes, exercise, massage).
d. Therapy utilizing nude body imagery exercises before a mirror with the spouse and sensate focus have proved particularly useful.
e. Usually the use of a prosthesis during intercourse psychologically perpetuates denial of surgery and the loss of the breast; however, if the prosthesis allows the woman to engage in sexual activity, it is temporarily encouraged.
f. Intercourse should be encouraged as soon as the woman is physically able after surgery (about one week postoperatively).

D. Diseases Commonly Affecting Sexuality
  1. Cardiac Disease Following Infarct (Hackett & Cassem, 1973; Hellerstein & Friedman, 1970; Kavanaugh & Shephard, 1977; McLane et al., 1980; Stein, 1977; Ueno, 1963).
     a. The majority of patients report anxiety and depression within the first year and after an anniversary reaction to the infarct.
     b. Almost all couples fear recurrent myocardial infarction (MI) and need specific educational counseling to prevent sexual dysfunction.
     c. The rise in heart rate, blood pressure, and O_2 consumption during intercourse post-MI has been shown to be no greater than that of walking briskly for a block.
     d. Most studies, unless congestive heart failure (CHF) or unstable angina interfere, demonstrated the safety of resuming sexual intercourse with an accustomed spouse four to six weeks post-MI.
     e. Deaths during coitus are a rarity, accounting for only 0.6% of all sudden deaths reported. Of this 0.6%, 80% occurred during intercourse with an extramarital partner.
     f. In a study of patients following their myocardial infarct, 60% of the men reported erectile difficulties and one-third reported premature ejaculation. Women following infarct reported more problems with orgasmic dysfunction than normal female controls.
     g. The therapist is aware not only of the above psychological issues, but also of the effect of cardiovascular drugs on sexual functioning.
  2. Vascular Disease—Strokes (Bray, DeFrank, & Wolfe, 1981)
     a. The majority of stroke survivors maintain consistent levels of sexual desire; however, most experience sexual dysfunction following a stroke.

b. Right hemiplegics often have problems with aphasia and apraxias. There may be problems with mood, memory, emotional lability, and judgment that may affect sexual functioning.
   c. Stroke affects communication, and engenders fear of repeat stroke secondary to sexual activity. These issues need to be discussed with the couple.
   d. Sensate focus needs to be addressed to the nonaffected side because of decreased sensory input following stroke.
   e. Alternate modes of sexual expression need to be explored when coital activity is compromised. These may include masturbation, oral-genital contact, or penile substitutes such as dildos or vibrators.
3. Respiratory Disease (Kass, Updegraft, & Muffly, 1972)
   a. Sexual dysfunction is usually secondary to psychological conflict in males who have conflict over stereotypically masculine roles related to issues of passivity and dependency.
   b. For patients with chronic obstructive pulmonary disease, use of low-flow portable oxygen and sexual positions that avoid compression of the chest wall, along with sexual counseling, are effective.
   c. Presexual use of bronchodilators or intermittent positive pressure breathing with postural and pulmonary toileting may prevent coughing episodes associated with exertion.
4. Endocrine Disease (Ellenberg, 1980; Kolodny, 1971; Kolodny, Kahn, Goldstein, & Barnett, 1974; Krosnick & Podalsky, 1981; Renshaw, 1979a, 1985)
   a. One-quarter of males under the age of 40 with diabetes have impotence uninfluenced by adequate medication or control of the diabetes.
   b. Fifty percent of females with a 20-year history or more of diabetes experience increasing sexual dysfunction. Ellenberg noted preservation of orgasmic ability in women with diabetes of long duration.
   c. Many diabetic men know that impotence may be a permanent complication of their disease, and resulting anxiety can cause dysfunction. It is wrong to assume that all diabetic patients with erectile impotence have impotence due to diabetes.
   d. Renshaw (1985) noted that psychogenic overlay in diabetic men is frequently overlooked. She noted that 26 of 27 diabetic men on insulin for 15 to 17 years recovered from the secondary impotence in 2 to 7 weeks with sexual therapy.
   e. Nocturnal penile tumescence (NPT) laboratory monitoring is

expensive, costing up to $1,500 per patient. A Snap-Gauge is an inexpensive (approximately $15.00) at-home test to measure NPT. At bedtime the patient places a velcro band around the base of the penis. The band has three plastic connector elements that snap sequentially as penile circumference increases during an erection. If all the elements have been broken by morning, a full girth erection is presumed to have occurred. Critics of the Snap-Gauge say results of the device can be incorrectly interpreted. They note that a momentarily rigid phallus may not be sufficient for intercourse.

5. Renal Disease (Milne, Golden, & Fibus, 1977–1978; Levy, 1979)
    a. Forty-five percent of patients with renal disease who were undergoing hemodialysis were noted to have decreased potency.
    b. In chronic renal disease fatigue, anemia, and uremia usually cause decreased sexual desire.
    c. The source of diminished potency in uremic men appears to be related to the relationship between the pituitary and Leydig cells in the testes.
    d. Dialysis for kidney insufficiency does not usually lead to improved sexual functioning in males; however, following renal transplants many dysfunctional males report restoration of sexual function.
    e. Females with chronic renal failure and hemodialysis note sexual dysfunction related to psychological and social difficulties; they also experience some improvement in sexual functioning following kidney transplantation.
6. Rheumatoid Disease (Ehrlich, 1978; Ferguson & Fingley, 1979; Richards, 1980)
    a. Studies of patients with osteoarthrosis of the hip joint note that over one-half experience disruption of sexual functioning.
    b. Recent studies of the etiology of sexual dysfunction in patients with arthritis have focused less on psychoanalytic, and more on somatic, factors, such as muscle weakness, joint pain, stiffness, limitation of motion, deformities, fatigue, and the secondary effects of pharmacotherapy.
    c. Psychodynamic factors include diminished feeling of sexual attractiveness secondary to altered body image and decreased self-esteem associated with diminished capacity in employment, activities of daily living, leisure activities, and self-care skills.
    d. Diagnostic assessment of the arthritis patient should include pre- and postsymptom sexual frequency, level of the patient's

and spouse's sexual satisfaction, positional variety of sexual activity with relation to symptoms, patient's sexual attitudes and responsiveness to engaging in alternative forms of sexual activity.
   e. Treatment strategies include:
      (1) Timing—sexual activity to correspond with desired pattern of greatest energy and comfort.
      (2) Drugs—utilization of analgesics and muscle relaxants and avoidance of narcotics or steroids that may interfere with libido.
      (3) Position—permission to experiment with positions that enhance comfort and promote sexual enjoyment.
      (4) Permission—to experiment with sexual options and to communicate effectively and openly about what is mutually pleasurable.
      (5) Surgical consultation regarding procedures to decrease pain and improve mobility.
7. Cancer (Andersen, 1985; Lieber, Plumb, Gerstenzang, & Holland, 1976; Wise, 1978, 1983)
   a. The etiology of sexual difficulties in cancer patients is multicausal, including sexual factors, physical disruption following treatment, and psychosocial factors.
   b. The two most prevalent affective changes among cancer patients are anxiety and depression that interfere with sexual functioning.
   c. Seventeen to 25% of hospitalized cancer patients have been found to be clinically depressed.
   d. Anxiety and depression can inhibit sexual desire, and anxiety significantly affects excitement and orgasm.
   e. Other somatic factors, such as fatigue, general debilitation, shortness of breath with coughing, bleeding with intercourse, and pain can also cause sexual dysfunction.
   f. Surgical treatment of cancer that results in disfigurement usually alters body image and causes sexual dysfunction; also, other cancer treatment (e.g., estrogens, radiation) can affect secondary sexual characteristics and alter body image (e.g., gynecomastia, alopecia).
   g. Estimates of sexual dysfunction in colon and rectal cancers in men have ranged from 32% to 59% for sexual desire, from 28% to 76% for erectile difficulties, and from 66% to 86% for ejaculation disruption. Twenty-eight percent of women with similar cancers noted reduced desire, and 21% reported genital numbness or dyspareunia.

h. Regarding whether sex therapy techniques are useful for cancer-related sexual dysfunctions, Anderson (1985) noted that sexual information and counseling improved general adjustment and sexual functioning.
8. Ostomy (Delin, 1969; Delin & Perlman, 1971)
   a. Cancer patients undergoing colostomies experienced a decrease in their sexual activity ranging from 38% to 75%.
   b. Men with colostomy had significantly greater disruption in their sexual activity than nonstoma surgical male patients, whereas women with colostomy compared with nonstoma women showed no significant differences in the magnitude of sexual dysfunction.
   c. Patients invariably fantasized that the ostomy adversely affected their relationship with their sexual partner.
   d. Peer counseling provided by ostomy associations has proven to be of considerable value in allaying fears and preserving sexual functioning.
   e. Some authors note that coital practice and frequency among patients with ileostomies do not differ from that of the general population.

V. Drugs and Sexual Dysfunction
(Abel, 1980; Kaplan, 1974; Medical Letter, 1980a,b, 1984; Papadopoulos, 1980; Segraves, 1977; Van Arsdalen & Wein, 1984)

Most reports of sexual dysfunction caused by drugs are clinical case reports with few controlled studies. Drugs interfere with the human sexual response by affecting desire, erection, ejaculation, and orgasm in men and decreased desire or orgasmic dysfunction in women. It is often difficult to differentiate pharmacological causes of sexual dysfunction from those related to psychosocial or disease etiologies.

A. Antihypertensive Drugs
   1. Diuretics are usually the first agent chosen to manage hypertension, and sexual side effects are minimal. Thiazides may occasionally inhibit vaginal lubrication. Spironolactone, however, can cause sexual dysfunctions, including impotence, painful gynecomastia, and menstrual abnormalities attributed to endocrine dysfunction.
   2. Adrenergic Inhibiting Drugs
      a. Rauwolfia alkaloids (reserpine)—10% of patients developed depression, which can affect sexual desire.

b. Guanethidine (Ismelin), a neurotransmitter depleter, caused ejaculatory impairment in 52% of patients and impotence in 31% of patients.
c. Methyldopa and clonidine—central sympatholytics, cause changes in potency, libido, and ejaculation.
d. Prazosin—blocks vascular postsynaptic alpha receptor and has been shown to cause the least sexual dysfunction.
e. Phenoxybenzamine—an alpha-adrenergic blocker. In some studies failure of ejaculation has been found; however, potency and orgasm were left intact.
f. Propranolol and metoprolol—beta-adrenergic blockers have been used as antianginals and anti-arrhythmics as well as antihypertensives. At first noted to rarely interfere with sexual functioning, propranolol has recently been shown to contribute to loss of libido and impotence in 7.4% of patients.
g. Hydralazine and minoxidil vasodilators have been implicated in some cases of impotence but are among the least likely to produce sexual dysfunction.

B. Antidepressant Drugs
1. Penile erection is primarily under parasympathetic control and is thought to be disrupted at the cholinergic and perhaps the alpha-adrenergic receptor sites.
2. Tertiary tricyclics, such as amitriptyline and imipramine, have greater sedative and anticholinergic side effects and cause more erectile and ejaculation problems than secondary amine tricyclics, such as nortriptyline and desipramine. However, diminished libido causing sexual dysfunction is usually improved with pharmacological improvement of depression.
3. Secondary amine tricyclic antidepressants are usually of first choice in the elderly because they have fewer muscarinic and sedative effects than the tertiary amines.
4. If impaired erection persists after switching from a tertiary to a secondary amine tricyclic, Pollack and Rosenbaum (1987) have noted improvement with the use of bethanechol 10 mg p.o. tid.
5. Priapism has been associated with the use of trazodone; it requires stopping the drug immediately and referral for urological consultation (Medical Letter, 1984).
6. Anorgasmia has been associated with heterocyclics and particularly with MAO inhibitors. Sovner (1984) has noted that central serotonergic mechanisms may be responsible for tricyclic anorgasmia. He has successfully used cyproheptadine (serotonin

antagonist) 4 mg Q.A.M. to treat anorgasmia associated with nortriptyline. Remission of anorgasmia has been known to follow after switching to less serotonergic drugs, for example, from amitrityline to desipramine.
C. Antipsychotic drugs—phenothiazines, thioxanthenes, and butyrophenones—all have been associated with some sexual dysfunction. Drugs with high sedative and anticholinergic activity have been associated with a higher prevalence of sexual dysfunction.
D. Antianxiety agents act as CNS depressants and can diminish sexual desire. However, if anxiety significantly interferes with the excitement and orgasm phases, the use of antianxiety agents may improve sexual functioning.
E. Sedative-Hypnotics and Alcohol (Abel, 1980; Munjack, 1979)
  1. Act as CNS depressants and inhibit sexual desire.
  2. However, in small amounts alcohol decreases anxiety and may enhance sexual desire.
  3. Prolonged alcohol use in males decreases testicular testosterone secretion, leading to diminished sexual desire. Continued alcohol abuse can lead to permanent liver damage with reduction of estrogen metabolism, increased plasma estrone, and plasma prolactin levels that cause feminization characteristics (gynecomastia, hair and skin changes) in males as well as testicular atrophy, decreased androgen, and permanent impotence.
F. Miscellaneous drugs associated with sexual dysfunction include cimetidine, clofibrate, digoxin, estrogens, indomethacin, lithium, methysergide, metoclopramide, metronidazole, and phenytoin (Van Arsdalen & Wein, 1984).

VI. Management of Sexual Dysfunction
(Crown & D'Ardenne, 1982; Cooper, 1981; Chapman, 1982; Glover, 1978; Hatch, 1981; Hawton, 1982; Kaplan, 1971; Levine, 1977)

It is beyond the scope of this chapter to discuss specific treatment of sexual dysfunction; however, general guidelines and indications for sexual therapy will be summarized.
A. General Guidelines for Management of Sexual Dysfunction in the Elderly
  1. Obtain appropriate sexual history, with particular attention to the effects of diseases and medications.
  2. Perform a complete physical, including a genital exam.
  3. Obtain consultation from the appropriate specialty.

4. Use graded approach to management; the approach, for example, described by Anon (1976)—PLISSIT model.
      P = Permission giving
      LI = Limited information
      SS = Specific suggestions
      IT = Intensive therapy
   5. The following are some additional general guidelines for all sexual dysfunctions.
      a. Reduce performance anxiety by initially prohibiting intercourse until improved sexual repertoire is possible.
      b. Encourage relaxation.
      c. Sensate focus to encourage increased receptivity to stimuli by having individuals engage in various forms of nongenital, nonerotic, physical pleasuring.
      d. Improve general communication between partners, particularly feedback about pleasuring.
      e. Set aside specific times for sexual relations that are free from pressures.
   6. For specific techniques (i.e., squeeze technique for premature ejaculation, positions for the medically ill, etc.), recommend authoritative general text, such as Masters and Johnson (1970), LoPiccolo and LoPiccolo (1978), Kaplan (1974), or Nadelson and Marcotte (1983).
B. Criteria for Deciding When to Refer Patients for Sex Therapy (Chapman, 1982)
   1. Absence of physical problem (e.g., infection, drug side effects).
   2. Absence of other primary problem (e.g., drug abuse, depression).
   3. Presence of bonafide sexual dysfunction in one or both partners (as defined in DSM-III-R).
   4. Presence of "therapy positive factors" (i.e., belief that therapy "works").
   5. Absence of interfering situational events (e.g., crisis, death in the family).
   6. Presence of a fairly adequate relationship between partners.
      a. Absence of, or arrest of, significant individual psychopathology.
      b. A conditional commitment between partners is established and clear.
      c. A basic repertoire of communication skills is present.
      d. "Relationship-relevant" material is not being excessively withheld.
      e. Mutually compatible life and relationship goals are present.

REFERENCES

Abel, E. L. (1980). A review of alcohol's effects on sex and reproduction. *Drug Alcohol Depend*, 5:321-332.
Abt, V., McGurrin, M. C., & Heintz, L. (1978). The impact of mastectomy on sexual self-image, attitudes, and behavior. *J Sex Education and Therapy*, 4(2), 43-46.
American Psychiatric Association. (1987). *Diagnostic and statistical manual of mental disorders* (3rd edition, revised). Washington, DC: American Psychiatric Press.
Andersen, B. (1985). Sexual functioning morbidity among cancer survivors. *Cancer*, 55, 1835-1842.
Anon, J. S. (1976). *The behavioral treatment of sexual problems: Brief therapy*. New York: Harper & Row.
Bengtson, V. L., Cuellar, J. B., & Ragan, P. K. (1977). Stratum contrasts and similarities in attitudes toward death. *J of Gerontology*, 32(1), 76-88.
Bray, G. P., DeFrank, R. S., & Wolfe, T. L. (1981). Sexual functioning in stroke survivors. *Arch Phys Med Rehabil*, 62, 286-288.
Burnap, D. W., & Golden, J. S. (1967). Sexual problems in medical practice. *Medical Education*, 42, 673-680.
Butler, R., & Lewis, M. (1976). *Sex after sixty: A guide for men and women in their later years*. New York: Harper & Row.
Carr, B. R., & MacDonald, P. C. (1985). The menopause and beyond. In R. Andres, E. L. Bierman, & W. R. Hazzard (Eds.), *Principles of geriatric medicine* (pp. 325-336). New York: McGraw-Hill.
Chapman, R. (1982). Criteria for diagnosing when to do sex therapy in the primary relationship. *Psychotherapy: Theory, Research and Practice*, 19(3), 359-367.
Cooper, A. J. (1981). Short-term treatment in sexual dysfunction: A review. *Comprehensive Psychiatry*, 22(2), 206-207.
Crown, S., & D'Ardenne, P. (1982). Symposium on sexual dysfunction: Controversies, methods, results. *BJ Psychiatry*, 140, 70-77.
Dagon, E. M. (1983). Aging and sexuality. In C. Nadelson & D. Marcotte (Eds.) *Treatment interventions in human sexuality* (pp. 357-375). New York: Plenum.
Dlin, B. (1969). Psychosexual response to ileostomy and colostomy. *Amer J Psychiat*, 126, 374-381.
Dlin, B., & Perlman, A. (1971). Emotional response to ileostomy and colostomy in patients over the age of 50. *Geriatrics*, 26, 112-118.
Ehrlich, G. (1978). Sexual problems in arthritis. In A. Comfort (Ed.), *Sexual consequences of disability* (pp. 61-84). Philadelphia: Stickley.
Ellenberg, M. (1980). Sexual function in diabetic patients. *Annals of Internal Med*, 92(2), 331-333.
Ellis, W. J., & Grayhack, J. T. (1963). Sexual functioning in aging males after orchiectomy and estrogen therapy. *J Urology*, 89, 895-899.
Ervin, E. V. (1973). Psychological adjustment to mastectomy. *Medical Aspects of Human Sexuality*, 7, 42.

Ferguson, K., & Fingley, B. (1979). Sexuality and rheumatic disease: A prospective study. *Sexuality and Disability, 2,* 130-138.

Finkle, A. L. (1978). Genitourinary disorders of old age: Therapeutic considerations including counseling for sexual dysfunction. *J Am Geriatric Soc, 10,* 453-458.

Finkle, A. L., & Prian, D. V. (1966). Sexual potency in elderly men before and after prostatectomy. *JAMA, 196,* 139.

Finkle, J. E. (1975). Encouraging preservation of sexual function after prostatectomy. *Urology, 6,* 697-702.

Frank, D. (1978). Mastectomy and sexual behavior. *Sexuality and Disability, 1.*

Furlow, W. L. (1980). Sexual consequences of male genitourinary cancer: The role of sex prosthetics. *Frontiers of Radiation Therapy and Oncology, 14,* 104-107.

Glowacki, G. (1978). *Postmenopausal GYN problems in the geriatric patient.* New York: H. P. Publishing Company.

Gordan, G. S., & Vaughan, C. (1977). The role of estrogens in osteoporosis. *Geriatrics, 39,* 142-148.

Griffith, E. R., & Treischmann, R. B. (1983). Sexual dysfunctions in the physically disabled. In C. Nadelson & D. Marcotte (Eds.), *Treatment interventions in human sexuality* (pp. 241-277). New York: Plenum.

Gurian, B. S. (1986). The myth of the aged as asexual: Counter transference issues in therapy. *Hosp Comm Psychiatry, 37*(4), 345-346.

Hackett, T. P., & Cassem, N. H. (1973). Psychologic adaptation to convelescence in myocardial infarction patients. In J. P. Naughton & H. K. Hellerstein (Eds.), *Exercise testing and exercise training in coronary heart disease.* New York: Academic Press.

Hart, M., Roback, H., Titler, B., Weitz, L., Walston, B., & McKee, E. (1978). Psychological adjustment of non-patient homosexuals: Critical review of the research literature. *J Clin Psychiat, 39,* 604-608.

Hatch, J. P. (1981). Psychophysiological aspects of sexual dysfunction. *Arch Sex Behav, 10,* 49-64.

Hawton, K. (1982). Symposium on sexual dysfunction: The behavioral treatment of sexual dysfunctioning. *Br J Psychiatry, 141,* 94-101.

Hellerstein, H. K., & Friedman, E. H. (1970). Sexual activity in post-coronary patients. *Arch Internal Med, 125,* 987-999.

Herr, H. W. (1979). Preservation of sexual potency in prostate cancer patients after I^{125} implantation. *J Amer Gerontological Society, 27,* 17-19.

Hogan, D. R. (1978). Effectiveness of sex therapy. In J. Lo Piccolo & L. Lo Piccolo (Eds.), *Handbook of sex therapy* (pp. 57-85). New York: Plenum.

Jackson, P. (1979). Sexual adjustment to hysterectomy and the benefits of a pamphlet for patients. *NZ Med J, 90,* 471-472.

Jaffe, L. (1974). Sexual problems of the terminally ill. In H. L. Gochros & J. S. Gochros (Eds.), *The sexually oppressed.* New York: Association Press.

Jonas, P. (1983). Post prostatectomy impotence in elderly patients. *Geriatrics, 38*(9), 113.

Kaplan, H. S. (1971, June). Sexual patterns at different ages. *Medical Aspects of Human Sexuality,* pp. 20-23.

Kaplan, H. S. (1974). *The new sex therapy: Active treatment of sexual dysfunctions.* New York: Brunner/Mazel.

Kavanaugh, T., & Shephard, R. (1977). Sexual activity after myocardial infarction. *Canadian Med Assn J, 116*(11), 1250–1253.

Kelly, J. (1977). The aging male homosexual: Myth and reality. *Gerontologist, 17*(4), 328–332.

Kimmel, D. (1978). Adult development and aging: A gay perspective. *J of Social Issues, 34*(3), 113–130.

Kinsey, A. C., Pomeroy, W. B., & Martin, C. E. (1948). *Sexual behavior in the human male.* Philadelphia: Saunders.

Kinsey, A. C., Pomeroy, W. B., & Martin, C. E. (1953). *Sexual behavior in the human female.* Philadelphia: Saunders.

Kolodny, R. C., Kahn, C. B., Goldstein, H. H., & Barnett, D. (1971). Sexual dysfunction in diabetic females. *Diabetes, 20,* 557–559.

Kolodny, R. C., et al. (1974). Sexual dysfunction in diabetic men. *Diabetes, 23,* 306–309.

Koss, I., Updegraff, K., & Muffly, R. (1977). Sex in chronic obstructive pulmonary disease. *Medical Aspects of Human Sexuality, 6,* 32–42.

Krosnick, A., & Podalsky, S. (1981). Diabetes and sexual function: Restoring normal activity. *Geriatrics, 36*(3), 92–100.

Levy, N. (1979). The sexual rehabilitation of the hemodialysis patient. *Sexuality and Disability, 2*(1), 60–65.

Lieber, L., Plumb, M. M., Gerstenzang, M. L., & Helland, J. (1976). The communication of affection between cancer patients and their spouses. *Psychosomatic Med, 38,* 379–389.

LoPiccolo, J., & LoPiccolo, L. (1978). *Handbook of sex therapy.* New York: Plenum.

Madorsky, M., et al. (1976). Effect of benign prostatic hypertrophy on sexual behavior. *Medical Aspects of Human Sexuality, 10,* 8–22.

Masters, W. H., & Johnson, V. (1966). Geriatric sexual response in the aging female and the aging male. *Human sexual response* (Chapters 15 and 16). Boston: Little, Brown.

Masters, W. H., & Johnson, V. (1970). *Human sexual inadequacy* (Chapters 12 and 13). Boston: Little, Brown.

McGuire, L. S., Guzinski, G. M., & Holmes, K. K. (1980). Psychosexual functioning in symptomatic and asymptomatic women with and without vaginitis. *Am J Obstet and Gyncol, 137,* 600–603.

McLane, M., Krop, H., & Mehta, J. (1980). Psychosexual adjustment and counseling after myocardial infarction. *Annals of Internal Med, 92,* 514–519.

Medical Letter on Drugs and Therapeutics (1980a). Drugs that cause sexual dysfunction, *22,* 108.

Medical Letter on Drugs and Therapeutics (1980b). Drugs that cause sexual dysfunction, *22,* 572.

Medical Letter on Drugs and Therapeutics (1984). Priapism with trazodone (Desyrel), *26,* 35.

Milne, J., Golden, J. S., & Fibus, L. (1977/78). Sexual dysfunction in renal

failure: A survey of chronic hemodialysis patients. *Int J Psychiat in Med*, 8(4), 335-345.
Munjack, D. J. (1979). Sex and drugs. *Clinical Toxicology*, 15(1), 75-89.
Nadelson, C. R. (1977). Emotional aspects of symptoms, functions and disorders of women. In G. Usden (Ed.), *Psychiatric medicine* (pp. 334-397). New York: Brunner/Mazel.
Nadelson, C., & Marcotte, D. (1983). *Treatment interventions in human sexuality*. New York: Plenum Press.
Papadopoulos, C. (1980). Cardiovascular drugs and sexuality. *Arch Int Med*, 140, 1341-1345.
Pfeiffer, E., (1974). Sexuality in the aging individual. *J Amer Geriatric Soc*, 22(11), 481-484.
Polivz, J. (1974). Psychological reactions to hysterectomy: A critical review. *Am J Obstetrics and Gynecology 118*, 417-426.
Pollack, M. H., & Rosenbaum, J. F. (1984). Management of antidepressant-induced side effects: A practical guide for the clinician. *J Clin Psychiat.*, 48(1), 3-8.
Renshaw, D. C. (1979a). Diabetic impotence—inevitable or imposed. Part I. *Br J Sexual Med*, 6:48.
Renshaw, D. C. (1979b). Diabetic impotence—inevitable or imposed. Part II. *Br J Sexual Medicine*, 6, 35.
Renshaw, D. C. (1985). Sex, age, values. *J Amer Geriatrics Soc*, 33(9), 635-643.
Richards, J. S. (1980). Sex and arthritis. *Sexuality and Disability*, 3, 97-104.
Segraves, R. T. (1977). Pharmacological agents causing sexual dysfunction. *J Sex Marital Ther*, 3, 157-176.
Sovner, R. (1984). Treatment of tricyclic antidepressant-induced orgasmic inhibition with cyproheptadine. *J Clin Psychopharmacol*, 4, 169.
Stein, R. A. (1977). The effect of exercise training on heart rate during coitus in the post myocardial infarction patient. *Circulation*, 55, 738-739.
Tollison, C. D., & Adams, H. E. (1979). *Sexual disorders: Treatment, theory, research*. New York: Gardner Press.
Ueno, M. (1963). The so-called coition death. *Japanese J. of Legal Med.*, 17, 535-541.
Van Arsdalen, K. N., & Wein, A. J. (1984). Drug induced sexual dysfunction in older men. *Geriatrics*, 39(10), 63-70.
Verwoerdt, A. (1969, February). Sexual behavior in senescence. *Geriatrics*, pp. 137-154.
Walsh, P. D., & Mostwin, J. L. (1984). Radical prostatectomy and cystoprostatectomy with preservation of potency. Results using a new nerve sparing technique. *Br J Urology*, 56, 694-697.
Wise, T. N. (1978). Sexual functioning in neoplastic disease. *Medical Aspects of Human Sexuality*, 12, 16-31.
Wise, T. N. (1983). Sexual dysfunctioning in the medically ill. *Psychosomatics*, 24(9), 787-805.

Witkin, M. (1975). Sex therapy and mastectomy. *Journal of Sex and Marital Therapy*, 1.

Ziel, H. K., & Finkle, W. D. (1975). Increased risk of endometrial carcinoma among users of cojugated estrogens. *NEJM, 23*, 1187.

ADDITIONAL READINGS

Asken, M. J. (1975). Psychoemotional aspects of mastectomy: A review of recent literature. *Am J Psychiatry, 132*, 56–59.

Cole, N. J. (1980). Drugs that influence sexual expression. *Consultant*, March, 183–291.

de Beauvoir, S. (1972). *The coming of age*. New York: G. P. Putnam.

Fine, H. L. (1974). Sexual problems of chronically ill patients. *Medical Aspects of Human Sexuality*, October, 137–138.

Kirkpatrick, J. R. (1980). The stoma patient and his return to society. *Frontiers of Radiation Therapy and Oncology*, 14.

Laner, M. R. (1978). Growing older male: heterosexual and homosexual. *The Gerontologist, 18*, 496–501.

Levine, S. B. (1977). Marital sexual dysfunction: Female dysfunction. *Annals of Internal Med, 86*, 588–597.

Leviton, D. (1978). The intimacy/sexual needs of the terminally ill and widowed. *Death Education, 2*, 261–280.

Neugarten, B., & Datan, N. (1974). The middle years. In S. Arieti (Ed.), *American Handbook of Psychiatry* (2nd ed.) (Vol. 1) (pp. 592–608). New York: Basic Books.

Pfeiffer, E. (1977). Determinants of sexual behavior in middle and old age. *J Amer Geriatric Soc, 20*(4), 151–158.

Raphael, S., & Robinson, M. (1981). Lesbians and gay men in later life. *Generations*, VI(1). Quarterly J Western Gerontological Society.

Reyendes, B. B. (1981). Triple whammy: Aging, sexuality and terminal illness. *Generations*, VI, No. 1, Quarterly J of the Western Gerontological Society.

Veath, J. (1980). *Body image, self-esteem and sexuality in the cancer patient*. Basel: S. Karger.

Wright, J. (1977). The treatment of sexual dysfunction: A review. *Arch Gen Psychiat, 34*, 881–890.

4
Medical Aspects of Aging

Raymond Vickers

I. Introduction

Eighty percent of the elderly have at least one chronic medical disease, so knowledge about important underlying medical illness is critical for the geriatric psychiatrist. Patients receiving geropsychiatric care often need treatment for their other illnesses; some of these treatments may be affected by the psychiatric condition or its therapy. Many medical illnesses and medications used to treat them can cause delirium, depression, anxiety, or psychosis in elderly patients, but certain disorders predictably have an impact on the mental status or psychiatric treatment; they are discussed in this section. The following guidelines are useful in recognizing patients who may have an organic basis to their psychiatric illness:
A. The presence of unexplained concomitant physical problems.
B. Unusual presentations, for example, atypical age of onset; lack of expected family history; symptoms that are out of proportion to expectations.
C. Poor response to psychiatric treatment.
D. Abrupt personality change, followed by blatant psychopathology.

II. Infections
(Gleckman & Ganz, 1983)

The presenting symptoms of many infectious diseases may resemble anxiety or psychoneurotic reactions. Infectious diseases also are included in the differential diagnosis of delirium, depression, and psychosis in the elderly.

A. Infections with presenting symptoms resembling psychogenic reactions may result in a patient being seen for psychiatric evaluation before the infection is manifest. Most of these conditions can be readily recognized if their existence is kept in mind.
   1. Tuberculosis (Stead & Dutt, 1985) reaches its peak rate in the elderly; 30% of new cases occur in persons over 65. It may present without respiratory symptoms, and constitutional signs may only include irritability, depression, and a marked need for rest. About 20% of old people in several series of nursing home admissions have a positive PPD; this usually is the immunological marker of prior infection, long since healed, but it can indicate miliary or extrapulmonary infection as well as reactivated pulmonary tuberculosis, even in the presence of a quiescent chest x-ray. In environments where a positive PPD rate is higher in the base population, this means a loss of reactivity due to aging (anergy). Sputum culture is indicated in the presence of suggestive symptoms, as are serial x-rays when the patient might be vulnerable because of disease or drugs that threaten immunological defenses or the patient is confined in a psychiatric or long-term care institution. A number of recent epidemics have occurred in nursing homes.
   2. Tetanus (Shands, 1979), which is totally preventable by immunization, is tenfold more common among those over 60 than among teenagers, and the fatality rate is 25 to 50 times higher. In a fully alert patient with the pathognomonic presenting picture of painful stiff jaw and back, a search for the sweating, low-grade fever and tachycardia of tetanus should come before considering neuropsychiatric causes such as the tetanus-like dystonia that may result from neuroleptic overdosage. In those never protected, tetanus immunization can be initiated at any age; two 0.5 ml. subcutaneous injections are given six weeks apart, followed by another a year later. Boosters should be given at least each 15 years, and as often as each 5 years if penetrating injuries, fistuli, or decubiti occur. Tetanus immune globulin 250 units is indicated for treatment of dirty or deep wounds in the patient who has had less than two doses of toxoid.
   3. Herpes zoster (Harnisch, 1984) has an annual incidence of 1% or 2% in those over 80; the incidence over age 70 is five times that at 50. The risk is greater in those with cancer or those who have had immunosupressant therapy. The typical vesicular rash is distributed along a dermatome, and is preceded by four to five days of pain and fever. The pain is often sudden, severe, and may

occur without a rash (zoster sine herpete); such a patient may be suspected of malingering, especially the rare one with motor palsy. Diagnosis is usually clinical, but varicella-zoster virus (VZ) can be confirmed by Tzanck smear inclusions or VZ immunofluorescence of serum. The patient should be isolated, and the rash treated with ionic solutions. Some physicians use steroids in the early stages, but the practice is not generally recommended, especially in psychiatric patients, unless ophthalmic involvement occurs. Oral acyclovir has been used for severe cases, and seems to help in the early stages, but may not shorten the course. Tricyclics are often helpful for postherpetic neuralgia, which is especially common in the elderly; 75% of those over 75 have this complication.

B. Infectious diseases causing delirium and psychosis are often seen by a psychiatrist on referral, sometimes with a request for psychopharmacological control of symptoms. It is important to ensure that adequate diagnostic procedures and specific therapy are being undertaken in such patients, since symptomatic treatment alone may cover up a potentially fatal infection.

1. Gram-positive infections (Gleckman & Ganz, 1983) in the elderly may present with major changes in the mental status. Older patients can remain entirely free of the usual localizing symptoms, such as cough in pneumonia, headache in meningitis, the pain of an abscess, or valvular murmurs in endocarditis. When community-acquired, these infections tend to be caused by gram-positive organisms. Usually, however, constitutional signs occur, including fever, tachycardia, increased respiratory rate, or leukocytosis, but any of these may be present singly. Therefore, in elderly patients with rapidly developing mental syndromes and any one of these constitutional clues, chest films, sputum, urine and blood culture (and, when nuchal rigidity is present, a lumbar puncture) should not be delayed by attempts to control symptoms with psychoactive drugs.

2. Gram-negative septicemia (Esposito, Gleckman, & Cram, 1980) is more common in elderly males; the incidence is increased by the use of catheters, intravenous infusions, and cardiac prosthetics, especially in patients who are demented or cachectic. Gram-negative septicemia should be suspected in any such vulnerable patient who has symptoms of confusion or disorientation and unexplained fever for more than a week. Gravely ill patients present with hyperventilation and hypotension and may remain hypothermic, a combination always suggestive of

gram-negative shock. Patients with these progressive symptoms are often observed for several hours in the hope that localizing signs will develop; any resulting delays in taking blood cultures and initiating appropriate therapy may be reflected in a high mortality.

3. Herpes simplex encephalitis (Scheibel & Raczek, 1985) is rare but might be suspected in a febrile illness with mental changes and a negative workup for bacterial infection. In the elderly, onset may appear gradually as hallucinations, acute memory disturbance, or personality change following a few days of fever and sore throat. Subacute limbic encephalitis of later life is probably a variant and may present as amnesic-confabulatory psychosis in a patient with remote cancer. Lumbar puncture and tomography scan are often negative in these conditions, but EEG has been reported as always abnormal and therefore should be done on patients in whom the search for a bacterial cause of infection is negative. Only brain biopsy is conclusively confirmatory. Full recovery has been reported in patients receiving adenine arabinoside therapy.

4. Syphilis (Holmes, 1983) is relatively rare, but recognition is easy and treatment is important to halt otherwise permanent damage. Possibly acquired during a "midlife crisis," neurosyphilis may present in late life as psychosis, depression, dementia, or a subtle personality disorder. The diagnosis might be overlooked because unreliability characterizes the history; an Argyl Robertson pupil is difficult to confirm in a senile eye; and slurred speech, trophic changes, areflexia, ataxia, and sensory symptoms are all mimicked by aging and may not be accorded diagnostic significance. Serology is no longer included in the routine tests performed on admission in many hospitals, so it must be specifically ordered in the workup of elderly patients with neuropsychiatric symptoms. Over 20% of cases of tertiary syphilis have a negative VDRL, and even when a diagnostic serology is reported it may be mistaken as one of the 60% false positives expected in the elderly. A fluorescent treponemal antibody absorption test (FTA-ABS) or a treponema pallidum hemagglutination test (TPHA) is confirmatory in 100% of cases of tertiary syphilis, even in the elderly. Serological tests on the spinal fluid are needed for a diagnosis of neurosyphilis and for monitoring the response to antibiotic treatment. Since syphilis is one of the reversible causes of dementia, a search for its presence is justified in the workup of brain syndromes, despite the low incidence.

III. Cancer
(Peterson & Kennedy, 1979)

Malignancy is the second leading cause of death at all ages (20% of the total mortality). The incidence of malignancy increases with age through the 90th year, 50% of all cancers occurring in persons over 65 years of age. Knowledge about the special aspects of cancer in the elderly is thus important for all who work with this age group. Of additional interest to psychiatrists are symptoms of cancer that have a psychosomatic basis (Peterson & Perl, 1982). Advanced invasive and metastatic disease requires a team approach, such as the exemplary practices seen in many hospices. The geriatric psychiatrist should have a significant role with such a team, not only in ensuring that treatment is considerate of the special needs of the elderly and that therapeutic enthusiasm does not extinguish ethical propriety, but also to ensure that patients do not lack opportunities for emotional relief because of unconscious ageism on the part of the staff.

The first research team to study the psychological impact of cancer and its therapy was established as an area of scientific inquiry more than 30 years ago, and special problems were identified with each area of cancer (Sutherland, 1956).

Ten of the sites discussed below account for the majority of all cancer deaths in the elderly; five of these major sites are in the alimentary system. Several other neoplasms are described because they also cause psychiatric symptoms or because of the importance of routine screening for them.

A. Alimentary system cancers account for 35% of all malignant neoplasms in the elderly; there are two prognostic groups. The first, salvageable cancers, are those in which detection at an early stage is possible because of their proximity to orifices; and the five-year survival of patients treated when these cancers are still localized exceeds 80%. Delay in diagnosis is often due to fear and other psychological factors, or to lack of an assiduous search, rather than false-negative examinations. The role of the physician is primarily in prevention and case-finding. The second group is located away from orifices and requires instrumentation for visualization. Less than 25% are localized at discovery, and the remainder have a five-year survival of less than 5%. Here the physician's role is in the support system.

    1. Lip and oral cancers (Chiodo, Eigner, & Rosenstein, 1986) account for 3% of all new cancers; the incidence has doubled in 15 years. Seventy-five percent of deaths are in those 55 and older; most of these are cancers of the tongue. Associated with expo-

sure to alcohol (the greatest risk factor), tobacco, and irritants, almost all can be seen or felt by examination. Biopsies should be requested on all ulcerated or nodular lesions of the lip, tongue, and mouth that do not heal in two weeks.

2. Colorectal cancer (Stroehlein, Goulston, & Hunt, 1984) is the most fatal gastrointestinal cancer in late life, accounting for about a quarter of all tumor deaths. Half of the incidence is in those over age 60, one-third being between the ages of 70 and 80. Patients with adenocarcinomas in the localized stage would be usually salvageable, but early evidence of the presence of a tumor is frequently ignored or the changes rationalized as normal aging. Symptoms include stool frequency changes, constipation and colicky pain, bleeding, hemorrhoids, mucous discharge, and distension. Detection of occult blood, especially in patients with unexplained anemia, is critical. Many of the tumors can be felt on rectal examination; most can be seen at sigmoidoscopy. The American Cancer Society recommends that all persons over 40 should have a rectal examination and a stool occult blood test annually, a sigmoidoscopy every four years, and more often if family history is positive or polyps are found (Eddy, 1980).

3. Esophageal cancer has an average onset at age 60 to 65. It is the fifth commonest cancer of males (7%), occurs three times as frequently in black people as in whites, and is commonest in heavy drinkers and smokers. The initial symptom of organic dysphagia must be carefully distinguished from functional difficulties in swallowing often seen in anxiety states. Progressive dysphagia for solid food is always a pathological sign; and when accompanied by recent weight loss in a person over age 40, it should always be investigated. Esophagrams, endoscopy, and biopsy are commonly used for diagnosis. The terminal stages may be particularly distressing and often call for palliative radiotherapy, narcotics, and much support. Gastrostomy and esophageal shunts can be used to prolong life if this is what is desired by patients and their families.

4. Stomach cancer (Lawrence, 1986) was once more prevalent, but overall the incidence has fallen 50% in the last 50 years; it is now the seventh commonest cause of death from malignancy. The incidence is highest after age 50; in women it is 50% of that in men. Presenting symptoms are often vague and are similar to complaints often heard from older psychiatric patients—anorexia, weight loss, and postprandial pain in the epigastrium. Suspicious features that should suggest further investigation of such complaints include any recent change in the pattern of

dyspepsia, such as a less constant relation to meals or a specific distaste for meat. Vomiting and microcytic anemia are significant. Investigations should include an upper GI series and gastroscopy with brush cytology or biopsy. Alternatively, exfoliative cytology of blind lavage centrifugate may be utilized.

5. Pancreatic cancer is the second most common GI carcinoma. Its highest incidence, at age 60-70, has tripled in the last 50 years. Patients may have no GI symptoms and present with what resembles a primary depression or be referred for other psychiatric symptoms, such as anxiety or rage attacks. A persistent sense of impending doom has been reported. Suspicious features of an organic etiology include lability of symptoms and treatment resistance. When symptoms referable to the pancreas (pruritic jaundice, anorexia, and pain in the back) do occur, resectability is rarely possible. Diagnosis may be made by sonographically directed needle biopsy, axial tomography (CT scan), nuclear magnetic resonance, or selective angiography.

B. Other cancers: The remaining five leading sites of cancer causing death in the elderly lie outside the alimentary system. It is critical that they be "staged" at the time of diagnosis, because the prognosis at each stage may differ from that in younger patients and may lead to different treatment approaches. A conservative approach is reinforced by the slower advance of many cancers in the elderly and the coincidental hazards presented by other potentially fatal diseases. The elderly (and often significant others) often decline to undergo major procedures, and studies suggest that elderly patients tolerate pain and other symptoms of cancer better than do many younger persons. On the other hand, it has been found that older patients tolerate surgery better than was formerly believed, encouraging a more radical approach to treatment. Also, it has been well established that older people do not have an age-related intolerance to the toxic effects of antimitotic drugs in high dosage, as many oncologists believed in the past.

1. Lung cancer is now the most fatal neoplasm of both men and women over age 55. It can only be prevented by reducing carcinogenic inhalants. There is evidence that quitting smoking, even in late adult life, can reverse bronchial mataplasia (this prospect might suggest an opportunity for geriatric psychiatry to assist in a worthwhile cancer-prevention activity). Solitary small peripheral pulmonary "coin" lesions (Stage I) are usually detected by chance radiographically. Stage II lesions are larger and may have caused symptoms that led to investigation, but remain peripheral without intrathoracic or metastatic spread. Percutaneous

needle biopsy or the cytologic study of specimens obtained at bronchoscopy should distinguish between anaplastic tumors (round and oat-celled), for which chemotherapy has the best prognosis in patients over 70 (Clamon, Audeh, & Pinnick, 1982), and other carcinomas, for which surgical resection results in a five-year survival rate of 50%. More advanced lung cancer may require palliative surgery or irradiation, which is often effective in reducing vena caval and bronchial obstruction, hoarseness, and pain. Heavy doses of chemotherapy are often not indicated in this stage. A good knowledge of the pharmacology of effective pain relief is essential in caring for patients who have reached this stage (Foley, 1986).
2. Breast cancer (Moe, 1985), though the second commonest lethal cancer in women 33 to 74, is rarer and less lethal over age 75. However, the prospect of surgery represents no less a potent threat of disfigurement to the elderly than the younger woman. Covert discovery is not unusual and may be an unsuspected source of stress underlying psychological manifestations. Every woman should palpate her breasts monthly; all over age 50 are recommended to have a professional examination and xeromammography annually (American Cancer Society, 1982); most suspicious masses found should be biopsied. Radical mastectomy is not recommended as often today as previously, especially for elderly women. In localized growths, a lumpectomy may be considered, followed where appropriate by chemotherapy or local radiation therapy. Nonsteroidal antiestrogens have revolutionized therapy for estrogen-receptor-positive (ERP+) carcinoma in recent years, and even an ulcerating schirrhus mammary carcinoma in an elderly person may become stationary with hormonal therapy.
3. Prostatic carcinoma (Brendler, 1985) is the second commonest malignancy in American males and increases in incidence with age. Thus the routine digital rectal examination of elderly men is a necessary aspect of the complete physical examination. Death rates are highest in married whites aged 54–74. Stage A (occult) disease detected in a resected gland requires no treatment. Stage B disease (palpable as nodules by rectal examination) can be confirmed by perineal needle biopsy, and the prognosis for remission after surgery or radiation is good if spread can be prevented. Those men in whom prostatic cancer has spread beyond the gland locally (Stage C) or metastasized (Stage D) have a 40% five-year survival rate, which is less than half that in cases detected and treated earlier. Advanced disease is recog-

nized by pyelography, radionuclide bone scan, and fractionated serum acid phosphatase. Stage C disease and localized bone pain may be responsive to irradiation. Many oncologists now withhold therapy for Stage D disease (low-dose estrogen therapy or castration) until symptoms require it, since cardiovascular and psychological complications of these modalities may be significant.

4. Hematological malignancies are common in the elderly. Chronic leukemias (Silber, 1982), nodular well-differentiated lymphomas, Stage I and II Hodgkin's disease, and even some multiple myelomas may have a chronic course, can be followed conservatively, and need to be treated locally only as indicated for splenomegaly, anemia, and thrombocytopenia. Some patients develop delirium when they are in need of blood transfusions, but if confusion persists after transfusion, a neurological workup is warranted, since meningeal deposits cause similar symptoms. There is a recent trend in a few centers to treat the blast crises that terminate chronic leukemia and the rarer acute lymphoblastic leukemias of late life by intensive chemotherapy (Peterson & Perl, 1982); in the past, aggressive therapy of this kind was usually withheld from the elderly. The psychiatrist may have a role in the decision whether to recommend the risk, time, travel, and cost that such treatment entails.

5. Cerebral, subtentorial, and spinal cord tumors (Salcman, 1982) are rare; they increase in incidence toward old age but then fall. These are the malignancies most likely to escape accurate psychiatric diagnosis. Common modes of presentation include irritability and personality change. Mental dullness, delayed responses to questions, and somnolence are often prominent. Symptoms of astrocytoma may be present for many years. Frontal and temporal tumors may present as disturbed memory and mood; vague headache may occur. Tumors involving the limbic system may cause memory loss, delusions, assaultive behavior, and depression. Computerized axial tomography scans and nuclear magnetic resonance detect 90% of cerebral tumors; most of the remainder are found by electroencephalography and lumbar puncture. Gliomas and secondary metastases have a bad prognosis, despite treatment; other tumors may be resectable, with a full recovery, even in the elderly.

6. Miscellaneous neoplasms described below, although not the cause of a large number of deaths, achieve importance in old age because of unusual features or because of the frequency of psychiatric symptoms.

a. Endocrine tumors may present because of hormone disturbances or as masses. Carcinoid tumor or pheochromocytoma may produce profound depression or psychosis. Pituitary, parathyroid, and adrenal tumors may present with psychiatric symptoms because of an excess or deficiency of hormones. Multiple adenomatosis and ACTH-secreting oat-cell carcinoma of the lung may produce acute delirium. Thyroid cancer rarely is differentiated enough to produce hormonal and psychiatric effects. More commonly, the question of malignancy is raised in a patient with nodular goiter. A sudden change in a nodule or the onset of local symptoms may be a sign of malignant change and is an indication for needle biopsy or surgical excision. Rapidly fatal anaplastic thyroid carcinoma is more common in the very old, but all forms of thyroid cancer have a greater recurrence rate and mortality with increasing age. Ovarian carcinomas (Barber, 1986) cause more deaths in older women than cervical and endometrial cancers combined and have risen steadily in incidence over the past 40 years. The first symptoms are of a gastrointestinal nature, with bloating and flatulence in a woman who has not had them. They may cause bleeding, so it is important to investigate all unexplained postmenopausal bleeding. When an older woman is found to have a suspicious pelvic mass, it may be confirmed by ultrasonography; a tissue diagnosis can be obtained by peritoneoscopy.

b. Skin neoplasms (Robinson & Roenigk, 1980) are not often lethal but do cause disfigurement, loss of self-esteem, depression, and isolation in some individuals. Primary skin carcinoma is the commonest cancer in Caucasian people, and the incidence rises with age. The basal cell types invade local tissues, and squamous cell neoplasms metastasize. All require biopsy for diagnosis. Malignant melanoma is the leading cause of death from skin disease and is more aggressively malignant in late life. Although the five-year survival rate of those with treated lesions is gradually increasing, the incidence of new cases, as more sun worshippers enter the senium, is increasing epidemically. The following danger signs should point to the need for removal of suspected lesions.

(1) Change in area, surface characteristics, or elevation.
(2) Change in color, especially brown to black.
(3) Change in sensation, that is, itching or tingling.

c. Uterine and bladder cancers (Glowacki, 1983) are often signaled by bleeding. Cancer of the cervix (Nelson, Averette, & Richart, 1984) is relatively rare in women after age 60 who have normal cervical smears at that age. Women with Grade IIb or higher Papanicolaou smears or who report postmenopausal spotting or discharge require gynecological follow-up. Diagnosis is by biopsy. Surgical and radiation cure rates are high for early lesions. Endometrial cancer peaks in incidence after the sixth decade; it is twice as common as cervical or ovarian cancer, possibly because of the increased use of estrogens; it is less often fatal, probably because the frequency of early bleeding usually leads to a timely diagnosis by curettage. Bladder carcinoma is becoming more common in older men. Death rates increase five times each decade past 50. The sole symptom is painless hematuria.

IV. Endocrine, Nutritional and Metabolic Disorders

These are common disorders of the elderly that often present with psychiatric symptoms (Davis & Davis, 1983).

A. Thyroid diseases (Gilbert, 1986) occur much more commonly in later life than is generally recognized. Hypothyroidism occurs in 4% of the elderly. Hyperthyroidism has been seen in up to 4% of hospitalized geriatric populations. Both thyroid diseases have been incriminated as rare causes of dementia; each may be misdiagnosed as a psychiatric illness. Thyroid nodules are found in 4% of elderly, but usually are benign.

In all routine diagnostic evaluations of older persons, serum T_3, T_4, T_3RU, and TSH should be obtained. T_4 is transiently raised following admission in 33% of eumetabolic acute psychiatric patients; the cause is unknown. High T_4 is often seen in manic-depressive disease, especially after lithium. Normal T_4 and high T_3 are seen in the "T_3 toxicosis" often associated with multinodular goiter.

1. Hyperthyroidism in the older patient usually presents with the same classical neuromuscular, cardiac, or gastrointestinal symptoms as in the younger patient, but these symptoms are masked in 25% of cases in late life, especially by heart failure or infection. Commonly, hyperthyroidism mimics an anxiety state, but in 15% apathetic thyrotoxicosis resembles depression. Weight loss and tachycardia are common. Beta blocking drugs, which are taken by many older patients, also suppress thyroid symptoms, and a fatal thyroid storm may follow sudden withdrawal of blockade.

2. Acquired hypothyroidism (Klein & Levey, 1984) presents in a classic fashion (i.e. myxedema, weight gain, and bradycardia) in only one-third of older patients; in the majority debilitation, apathy, psychomotor retardation, pseudodementia, or depression are more common. Paranoid reaction and "myxedema madness" also occur, but true dementia and delirium are rare.

B. Diabetes affects 20% of the elderly population and its incidence is increasing, so it is inevitable that the geriatric psychiatrist will see diabetic patients.

  1. Uncomplicated diabetes (Goldberg, Andres, & Bierman, 1985) is often masked in the aged. Prior disease such as infection or dementia may overshadow its appearance; in fact, their treatment may increase the hyperglycemia itself (e.g., steroids, estrogens, thiazides). Psychological stress as well as acute disease may precipitate its onset. Early symptoms may first be mistaken as depressive, such as loss of energy and drive, fatigability, weight loss, or impotence. If polyuria leads to incontinence it may be misinterpreted as regression, as might pruritis vulvae also. Peripheral neuropathy and autonomic motor disturbances may resemble hysterical manifestations. Treatment decisions such as whether the patient can cope with self-administration of insulin or blood glucose monitoring may need prior psychological assessment. Noncompliance with a diet is a frequent expression of denial that may be amenable to psychotherapy.
  2. Hypoglycemia (Slovik, 1985) can occur during the treatment of diabetes because people miss meals or do not understand diets; it is most likely to follow attempts to "normalize" hyperglycemia with drugs or insulin. Some drugs used in the elderly potentiate hypoglycemia (e.g., β blockers, salicylates, and MAO inhibitors). Sulfonylureas may cause a hypoglycemia of slow onset, which presents as a florid psychosis or delirium. Prompt recognition of a low serum glucose may be life-saving in acute delirium.
  3. Ketoacidosis occurs in "insulin-dependent" (Type I) diabetes when the need for insulin exceeds the supply. While Type II (maturity-onset) diabetes, in which ketosis does not occur, is much commoner in the aged, Type I (previously known as "juvenile") occurs often enough to make ketoacidosis a cause that must be considered in the differential diagnosis of stupor in an aged patient. It may appear at any time and is rapidly fatal. Frequently precipitated by an infection (often occult), it may present as confusion or stroke. The blood glucose and acetone

level confirm the diagnosis; if recovery is to occur, rapid treatment is essential.
   4. Nonketotic hyperglycemic hyperosmolar coma (Cahill, 1983) may occur as the first indication of the onset of Type II diabetes after age 60. Neuropsychiatric symptoms rapidly worsen over a few days, ending in coma, which has a 50% fatality rate. Antihypertensives, CNS-active drugs, phenytoin, or cimetidine may precipitate the onset. Treatment includes expansion of intravascular volume, low-dose insulin administration, and potassium supplementation.
   5. Other complications of diabetes accumulate in the elderly.
      a. Arteriosclerosis is the cause of most deaths in the elderly. Diabetes may be a predisposing factor; its advance may be slowed by good control of hyperglycemia, but this is controversial. Some patients are able to accept "tight" control, others do better with a permissive approach; decisions are best made with knowledge about the patient's personality, supplemented by education about the disease. An example is the higher rate of gangrene in those diabetics who smoke compared with those who quit.
      b. Ophthalmic manifestations of diabetes are the leading cause of blindness in the United States today. Rehabilitation programs for the visually handicapped are enhanced by skilled psychiatric intervention.
      c. Sensory neuropathies may cause severe pain and lead to narcotic addiction. Motor mononeuropathy may mimic conversion reactions (e.g., wrist drop).
      d. Autonomic syndromes of diabetes (Gandhavadi, Rosen, & Addison, 1982) include postural hypotension, impotence, dysfunction of bladder and bowel, presbyesophagus, and gastroparesis; these autonomic syndromes may lead to diagnostic uncertainty in geriatric assessment. Autonomic pain syndromes including nonradicular dysesthesia, dyscrasia, dystrophy, and dysthymia may result in the mistaken conclusion that they are of purely functional origin because they do not follow the spinal dermatomes.
C. Hyperparathyroidism (Lafferty, 1981) peaks in incidence after age 55; 20% of patients are over age 65. The most common clinical presentation is with hypercalcemia and psychiatric symptoms resembling depression, which include lassitude, constipation, emotional lability, anxiety, and restlessness. Other manifestations may resemble personality disorder, delirium, dementia, or other psy-

chosis (Kleinfeld, Peter, & Gilbert, 1984). Somatic symptoms of neuromuscular, cardiovascular, renal tract, gastrointestinal, and joint disease may also occur. The diagnosis is often reached when an immunoreactive serum parathyroid hormone (PTH) level is obtained during the investigation of hypercalcemia found incidentally by routine serum screening. Circulating PTH levels rise a little with aging but are significantly increased in hyperplasia and adenoma of the gland. They are depressed in hypercalcemia due to causes other than primary hyperparathyroidism. In the elderly, the major differential diagnoses include squamous cell carcinomas, excessive Vitamin A and D consumption, and occasionally usage of thiazide.

D. Malnutrition (Foley, Libow, & Sherman, 1981) may result from apathy and poor judgment caused by depression, delirium, or dementia, but these conditions may be complications of malnutrition itself. There may be a background of socioeconomic causes and ignorance. Deficiencies can be associated with oral and dental problems or follow prolonged illness and immobility.
   1. Specific vitamin deficiencies may cause mental impairment during their course.
      a. Thiamine (Vitamin B_1) deficiency causes Korsakoff-Wernicke syndrome, with ocular palsies, nystagmus, ataxia, and global confusion in the acute stage, followed later by anterograde-retrograde amnesia, peripheral neuritis, and congestive cardiac failure. Most, but not all, patients give a history of alcoholism.
      b. Riboflavin-pyridoxin deficiency may cause depression and confusion with EEG changes; seborrheic dermatitis, cheilosis, and stomatitis also occur. It may also indicate prior excessive alcohol intake. B_6 supplements should not be given to patients with Parkinson's disease who are receiving levodopa because of interference with drug metabolism.
      c. Niacin deficiency causes pellagra (dementia, dermatitis, and diarrhea). Stomatoglossitis may also be seen. It is seen in protein malnutrition and loss of ileal function.
      d. Folic acid and B_{12} deficiencies (Crantz, 1985; Grinblat, 1985) are often seen separately, since the first occurs from lack of fresh foods and the latter in patients getting little meat. They can both cause reversible confusional syndromes, dementia, and macrocytic anemia (*vide infra*). Diagnosis should be by immunochemistry, since microbiological assay results do not correlate well with symptoms.

  e. Ascorbic acid deficiency, which is due to lack of fresh fruits and vegetables, causes lassitude, weakness, irritability, weight loss, myalgias, and bone pain, all readily mistaken for symptoms of a depressive disorder. Additionally, gingivitis, bleeding disorder, and delayed wound healing occur.
 2. Obesity is a special case of malnutrition that complicates the management of hypertension, heart failure, diabetes, emphysema, and arthritis. Psychiatric intervention where efficacious helps the patient to increase activity and motivation rather than to concentrate ineffectively on caloric restriction. Some obese individuals respond to cognitive inhibition or behavioral therapy. Other "overweight" individuals have a large body habitus and a heredity/endocrine predilection to fat accumulation. Psychotherapy with these patients helps them to accept themselves and not allow misdirected social pressures to cause depression or disruption of their social life.

E. Metabolic bone diseases are often viewed as being inevitable consequences of old age or are misdiagnosed as "arthritis" because the diagnostic challenge is avoided. Although little relief may be obtained in many cases, it is worthwhile to attempt diagnosis in order not to miss diseases where specific treatment is available. A detailed history implies respect for the patient's own concerns; a competent examination raises his confidence in the physician.
 1. Osteoporosis (Raisz, 1982), the loss of bone mass per unit volume, is almost universal in older women, less so in men. The pathologic physiology of the disease is not well understood, despite considerable research. Its treatment and possible prevention have been subject to some unsubstantiated claims. Major psychiatric concerns are:
  a. Caffeine, alcohol, and smoking all accelerate osteoporotic changes.
  b. The physical changes, which resemble the negative stereotype of the appearance of aged people, can be depressing to those afflicted by them.
  c. Pain, acute and chronic, is a problem and may lead to drug dependency.
  d. Estrogens may cause depression or, if used for the long term, may be hazardous.
 2. Osteomalacia (Barzel, 1983), the demineralization of bone, usually is caused by deficiency of Vitamin D in the diet, by malabsorption, or by a lack of sunlight, especially in those who are institutionalized. Low serum calcium phosphate and high

parathormone and alkaline phosphatase are characteristic. Diphenylhydantoin ingestion, acidosis, and renal diseases are rarer causes. Proximal limb pain and "waddling" (antalgic) gait are seen. Treatment is by Vitamin D therapy, with care to avoid hypercalcemia (and consequent psychiatric symptoms). Patients who fail to improve adequately on vitamin therapy may have both osteoporosis and osteomalacia.

F. Fluid and electrolyte disorders (Delmez, 1983) constitute a significant cause of psychiatric and medical disturbance in old age. Psychiatric symptoms include personality changes, hallucinations, delirium, and mania.

1. Volume depletion involves combined salt and water deficit more often than pure dehydration or hyponatremia. Prolonged diuretic therapy is a common etiology, but voluntary and involuntary deprivation also occur. Psychiatric consultation often is sought because the patient is delirious. Tranquilizers can make matters worse by further interfering with reality testing. Prompt infusions of normal saline are indicated, as well as medical and psychiatric treatment of the underlying etiologies.

2. Hyponatremia may occur with volume depletion as above, but also with a normal or increased volume (edema). When the serum sodium level falls below 125 mEq/l lethargy and behavior changes commonly occur. Continued sodium depletion can result in confusion, convulsions, and coma. Below 110 mEq/l irreversible brain damage is believed to take place. Combined sodium/volume depletion is treated by fluid replacement. Dilution hyponatremia seen with edema is usually insignificant; attempts to control it by fluid restriction are inappropriate and simply result in increased thirst.

   With a normal extracellular volume, low sodium may be due to renal failure or the syndrome of inappropriate secretion of antidiuretic hormone (SIADH.) Pain, emotional stress, psychiatric polydipsia, and drugs (e.g., neuroleptics, tricyclics, indomethacin, and chlorpropamide) can all be etiological factors in SIADH; and certain malignancies can mimic the effects of the hormone also. Treatment by strict restriction of fluid intake is effective and is preferable to saline infusions.

3. Hypokalemia is also common in the elderly. Initial symptoms may seem suggestive of psychotic depression, dementia, or other psychotic disorders. Treatment is by oral replacement (e.g., slow-release KCl). The causes of hypokalemia are:

   a. Diarrhea (including purgative abuse) and vomiting.

Medical Aspects of Aging

      b. Diuretic therapy.
      c. Dietary deficiency (the frail, the neglected, the anorexic).
  4. Hydrogen ion (pH) disturbances may produce mental status changes in acutely ill elderly patients.
      a. Respiratory alkalosis is seen in panic attacks, severe pain, and cirrhosis, as a result of hyperventilation, but rarely produces tetany. Treatment is by sedation.
      b. Metabolic alkalosis is seen after prolonged vomiting, especially in a patient with low potassium and volume depletion due to diuretics. Apathy and lethargy are seen, and, if the calcium is low, irritability and tetany. Treatment is by I.V. saline.
      c. Metabolic acidosis, seen in renal failure and diabetes, is characterized by weakness, malaise, vomiting, headache, and abdominal pain. Depressed diabetic patients who quit insulin may slip into acidosis without a mood change being noted.
      d. Respiratory acidosis produces drowsiness, stupor, and occasionally asterixis from hypercapnea. It may occur in oversedation, chronic lung failure, and cerebral disease; it is not unusual to see all these three etiologies together in one patient. Acidosis may occur suddenly if oxygen is being given at a high flow rate. Mechanical ventilation should be considered in the treatment.

V. Diseases of the Blood

These are significant sources of psychiatric symptoms, especially lethargy, depression, and confusion (Seligman, 1982).

A. Anemias in the elderly are common but easily overlooked (Coni, Davison, & Webster, 1980). They may be a good clue to the presence of other diseases. At times they lead to decompensation or have other grave effects, but frequently they can be corrected. Hemoglobin levels do not fall with healthy aging; the lower level of normal in males is 13g and 12g in females.
  1. Hypochromic anemia is usually due to iron deficiency. Before iron replacement is undertaken, blood loss should be seriously considered as a cause. If blood loss is ruled out, a trial on oral iron therapy would retrospectively confirm dietary deficiency if reticulocytes appeared and the hemoglobin level rose. Poverty, psychiatric illness, and fad diets may be to blame for dietary deficiency of iron. Failure to respond to iron should always be investigated carefully.

2. Megaloblastic anemias are usually due to either cobalmin or folate deficiency. The characteristic bone marrow changes are diagnostic.
    a. Pernicious anemia (PA) is the commonest cause of cobalmin (Vitamin B_{12}) deficiency anemia. It is diagnosed most frequently in aged persons with a positive family history. Parasthesiae, posterior column syndrome, and pyramidal signs may occur in pernicious anemia. The disease may present as dementia or delirium (Evans, Edelson, & Golden, 1983) without anemia. A low serum B_{12} level and a positive Schilling test can be diagnostic. The first injection of cobalmin should be followed by rising reticulocyte counts for confirmation. Lifetime treatment is necessary to avoid neurological damage as well as anemia.
    b. Folate anemia does not occur in most persons with folate deficiency, which is a common finding in the elderly. While mental symptoms may precede anemia in PA, they tend to follow anemia in folate and other associated vitamin deficiencies. To avoid myelopathy, it is important to ensure that any cobalmin deficiency concomitantly present is first corrected before folic acid is given.
    c. Anticonvulsant macrocytosis does not produce anemia and needs no treatment.
3. Hypoplastic anemia is often accompanied by other forms of marrow failure, with low platelet count and leukopenia. The etiology is often difficult to clarify; chlorpromazine and anticonvulsants have been incriminated infrequently; more often renal failure or cancer are responsible. Steroids are often given on the unproven assumption that an autoimmune etiology exists. Spontaneous recovery may occur.
4. Hemolytic anemia due to proven autoimmune reactions from medications, such as anticonvulsants, chlorpromazine, and chlordiazepoxide, is uncommon in the elderly. The only familial hemolytic anemia that seems to appear for the first time in later life is spherocytosis. Hemolytic anemias are recognized when the reticulocyte count and indirect bilirubin are raised and confirmed by a reduced tagged cell survival.

B. Neutropenia, a white cell count under 2,000/cu mm, may be seen in older individuals without any associated disease. However, it may be due to primary hematological disorder, such as preleukemia; to deficiencies of nutrients, such as folic acid; to chronic illness, such as cancer and renal disease; or to drugs. Drug-induced agranulocytosis is rare, but has significant medical and legal implications. It

often develops too quickly to be heralded by routine blood counts; the best warning is for the patient to report oral or pararectal sores to the physician.
C. Coagulation system disorders (Thompson, 1985) can occur at any age, but thromboembolism of both arteries and veins is a particularly frequent problem of the elderly.
   1. Defect of hemostasis must be suspected with any bleeding episode. If generalized or accompanied by dependent or mucosal petechiae, platelet and coagulation studies are indicated. Spontaneous benign petechiae and subcutaneous hemorrhages (devil's pinches) are often seen in the frail elderly and need no treatment. They may be mistaken as signs of physical abuse.
   2. Venous thrombosis develops in two-thirds of hospitalized patients aged 70–80; smoking increases the risk, but aspirin may reduce it. Without a high index of suspicion, thromboembolism usually is the first sign of thrombosis; often thromboembolism is missed. Therapy with heparin, though hazardous, may be indicated.
   3. Arterial embolism (Walshe, 1985) may occur anywhere, but constitutes a special hazard to the central nervous system. Large thrombi may come from the ventricular wall after myocardial infarction or the left atrium in fibrillation. Fibrillation associated with rheumatic heart disease is more likely to produce embolism than if from other causes. Massive embolic infarcts cause strokes; repeated microemboli cause transient ischemic attacks (TIAs) and may cause dementia. Prophylactic aspirin or dipyridamole may be indicated after TIAs.

VI. Cardiac
(Lindenfeld & Groves, 1982)

Diseases of the heart and blood vessels are the major source of medical morbidity in late life and contribute to psychiatric symptomatology in many ways. Slightly over half of deaths of those aged 65 to 74 in the Framingham study were due to cardiovascular disease.
A. Valvular heart disease in the aged commonly involves the mitral and aortic values.
   1. Rheumatic mitral disease (Caird, 1982) occurs in 2–4% of the elderly. Unrecognized or forgotten rheumatic fever in early life is the usual cause of the valvular damage. Half of elderly patients with mitral disease are asymptomatic, but 33% have fibrillation and 10% suffer embolism; either may be the cause of CNS complications. Most patients with symptoms of cerebrovascular

disease show left ventricular preponderence on the electrocardiogram; if a right preponderence is seen, especially with fibrillation, dyspnea and fatigue, or congestive failure, mitral stenosis may be present, and a chest film and echocardiography are indicated even in the absence of characteristic ausculatory findings. A timely mitral commissurotomy in such a patient might prevent a stroke.
2. Aortic valve insufficiency (Kotler, Mintz, Parry, & Segal, 1981) is the most common congenital or rheumatic valvular disease lasting into old age. Decompensation, which is unusual before the age of 50, is heralded by dyspnea and fatigue. Findings include a high-pitched dialastolic murmur along the left sternal border and a water-hammer pulse. X-ray and cardiogram show enormous hypertrophy. Aortic calcification suggests a syphilitic etiology and should prompt a further search for neurosyphilis.
3. Aortic stenosis (Santinga, Flora, Kirsch, & Baublis, 1983) is suggested by a harsh aortic systolic ejection murmur, but this is of little help in diagnosis or prognosis. However, a diminished aortic second sound and evidence of left ventricular hypertrophy are reliable signs. Stenosis may be calcific or hypertrophic; in both, the occurrence of exertional dyspnea, angina, and syncope are grave symptoms, as is congestive failure.
4. Mitral valve prolapse (Snyder, 1985) is a disease of older age groups in which the posterior leaflet undergoes mucoid degeneration and buckles in midsystole, giving a characteristic click and echocardiographic picture. Unusual behavior patterns may be seen, panic attacks may occur, and possibly transient cerebral ischemic attacks (TIA's) from microemboli.

B. Coronary artery disease (CAD) is the most frequent cause of death after age 50; it accounted for 30% of the cardiovascular deaths in the Framingham study.
1. Angina pectoris (Katz, 1986) is less common in older persons with CAD than in younger adults and is seen in less than 50% of those dying with the disease. Sometimes symptoms may not be reported because of cognitive defects. Symptomatic CAD is more likely to coexist with other causes of pain, such as aortic stenosis, hiatus hernia, arthritis, and cholecystitis, causing difficulty in diagnosis; a therapeutic trial of nitroglycerine may be helpful. Atypical syndromes, such as nocturnal and decubitus angina or diaphoresis, have a serious prognosis but are often unrecognized; they may result in a suspicion of functional disease and a referral for psychiatric evaluation. Interpretation of exercise stress testing of many elderly people is difficult because

of exhausting protocols and false-positive baseline changes; often, holter monitor and echocardiographic recordings are useful diagnostic adjuncts. The decision to have bypass surgery, based on cardiac catheterization, is often made arbitrarily, since there is controversy about the interpretation of outcomes in large published series that compare mortality after surgery with conservative management. Individual decisions may be assisted by appropriate psychological assessment of the patient's level of pain, lifestyle, and ability to cope with change.
2. Myocardial infarction (Rodstein, 1971) presented classically in the elderly less than 50% of the time in some series. Mental confusion and restless agitation occurred often enough to justify an ECG as part of the evaluation of elderly psychiatric patients; serial cardiac enzymes and noninvasive procedures also have a place in the workup of acute mental confusion. In the coronary care unit, the psychiatrist has a key role in the evaluation of confusion and other symptoms, reducing the stress of first encounters with hi-tech equipment, working with patients and families in life-sustaining decisions and with staff to reduce ageism and burnout.
3. Cardiac arrest (Moss, 1986) is the commonest cause of sudden unexpected death outside the hospital. It is due to cardiac standstill or ventricular fibrillation, usually caused by CAD. It often occurs in the stage of catechol release following exertion or emotion, rather than during the stress itself. All physicians should be able to recognize arrest instantly and to know cardiopulmonary rescuscitation technique. The ethical questions that surround the decision to use "do not rescuscitate" orders must be faced in geriatric facilities, and the psychiatrist has a significant role in the conduct of discussions about this with staff, patients, and their families (Gordon & Hurowitz, 1984).
   a. Signs of cardiac arrest at approximate points in time:
   Zero seconds: sudden pulselessness
   10 seconds: unconsciousness
   20 seconds: convulsions (may be absent)
   30 to 45 seconds: apnea
   60 seconds: pupils dilate
   4 minutes: irreversible brain damage
   b. Outline of cardiopulmonary resuscitation (CPR mnemonic):
   ABC: A blow to the chest (precordium), followed by:
   A: Airway maintenance
   B: Breathing assistance (artificial respiration), and
   C: Cardiac compression (monitor pulse)

4. Arrhythmias and conduction defects (Harris, 1982) increase in incidence with age. They are often poorly tolerated because they tend to cause disequilibrium of cardiac output and symptoms in target organs such as the brain. Intermittent arrhythmias may require holter monitoring to diagnose the cause of intermittent behavioral symptoms (Fleg & Kennedy, 1982). Arrhythmias of particular interest to psychiatry are:
   a. Atrial fibrillation at 60 to 100 beats per minute is often well tolerated in the elderly, but digoxin may be required to reduce higher rates. Conversion may prove to be difficult or impossible. Thyrotoxicosis may be the cause of fibrillation.
   b. Sick sinus syndrome or bradycardia-tachycardia, a cause of intermittent weakness, syncope, and vague neurotic complaints. Digitalis is contraindicated because of the danger of increasing the degree of block; a pacemaker is indicated.
   c. Atrioventricular block is commonly caused by digitalis and responds to reduction in dosage. If second or third degree or persistent, a pacemaker may be indicated. Complete heart block is a cause of intermittent confusional syndrome and is also likely to result in falls.
5. Infective endocarditis (Smith, 1986), if unrecognized, is usually fatal; autopsy data indicate that the diagnosis was not made during life in 50% of geriatric patients dying with the disease. Twenty-five percent of all cases occur after age 60, and the geriatric incidence appears to be increasing, possibly because of earlier diagnosis. Acute endocarditis has an onset in the aged with fever, myalgia, and arthralgia; cerebral or other embolism is the first sign in 40%. The commoner subacute form may present with anorexia, inanition, and malaise; often confusion, sterile meningitis, stroke, or coma cause hospitalization. The ideal plan to manage elderly admissions with anemia, undiagnosed fever, and valvular murmurs is to withhold antibiotics until blood cultures can be drawn. Mortality in treated cases increases with age and delay in diagnosis.
6. Hypertension (Applegate, 1986) is present in 40% of people over 65 in the United States, often resulting in heart failure, renal disease, and stroke. It is also associated with multiple infarct dementia. The successful control of blood pressure results in a demonstrable reduction in morbidity, but the drugs used for this purpose are also responsible for drug-induced depression or reversible dementia (Hale, Stewart, & Marks, 1984). Weight loss and salt reduction alone should be pursued where possible. Older hypertensives who do need drugs are often maintained on

diuretics and beta blockers. Recent work has suggested that after antihypertensive drugs have succeeded in maintaining a satisfactory level of blood pressure for several years, the pressure will remain down after medication withdrawal in over 40%.
7. Congestive cardiac failure usually has a gradual onset, but can be recognized by detection of weight gain and early symptoms. Patients usually complain of fatigue, anxiety, dyspnea, and edema. If pulmonary edema occurs it may be mistaken for a panic disorder. With sedentary patients the only symptoms may be impaired concentration and memory loss, but confusion may also occur. The commonest cause is CAD, but hyperthyroidism, anemia, arrhythmia, valvular disease, and pulmonary embolism should be considered. Diet, diuretics, and digoxin are the mainstays of therapy; however, since the latter are both potent causes of delirium and dementia, regular electrolyte monitoring and trial withdrawal of digoxin should often be considered in patients whose cardiovascular status has stabilized (Stults, 1982).

VII. Pulmonary Diseases

These are common and significant causes of medical morbidity in the elderly and complicate psychiatric disorders.
A. Pneumonia (Bartlett, 1985), termed "the old man's friend" by Osler, has an incidence and mortality that rises steeply with age. Some lung infiltration is found in 50% of x-rays of older people dying in hospitals; where radiology is not available, the diagnosis must be frequently missed. Among important causes of pneumonitis in the elderly, especially in the demented and those taking neuroleptics, is aspiration. Delirium, a very common feature of pneumonia, especially in Legionnaires' disease, is often the presenting symptom in the elderly, because cough, fever, pleurisy, and sputum may be absent. Common signs include tachypnea and general deterioration; cyanosis, hypotension, and tachycardia often indicate a grave prognosis. A chest film is indicated in any older patient with acute mental clouding and a respiratory rate of 25 per minute or over. Initial therapy should be determined by the results of a Gram stain of the sputum. It is wise to consider withholding sedatives and tranquilizers for the treatment of sudden delirium until pneumonia can be excluded, since they may compromise successful therapy.
B. Chronic obstructive lung disease (COLD) (Brown & Scharf, 1985) usually has an onset in earlier life as small airway disease due to

bronchitis, bronchiectasis, or asthma, especially in smokers, with persistant cough as the only symptom. Whether primarily a disease of bronchioles (chronic bronchitis) or of alveoli (emphysema), the pathological changes ultimately result in chronic airway obstruction. Agitation, paranoid behavior, and intermittent confusion may be seen in the later stages, because of hypoxemia and hypercapnea. The rehabilitation of patients with chronic pulmonary disability requires an interdisciplinary approach in which psychological input is critical. Relief may be experienced by the use of O_2, xanthines, and β_2-adrenergic drugs. Risks of therapy include loss of respiratory drive from high oxygen flows, drug dependency, and an atropine-like psychosis, especially when steroids are also used. Sedatives, which are respiratory depressants, are relatively contraindicated, as are beta blocker drugs, widely used in the elderly for treatment of angina and hypertension, because they increase bronchospasm. Monoamine oxidase inhibitors cannot be used to treat the pervasive depression often found in COLD if the patient is taking bronchodilators, because of the epinephrine-like action of the latter.

C. Pulmonary embolism (Brown & Scharf, 1985) causes 50,000 deaths a year; 90% are over age 50. Embolism is unsuspected during life in 50% of these. It is commonly associated with congestive heart failure, blood dyscrasia, obesity, decubitus, trauma, and cancer. The origin of the embolus is usually venous thrombosis of the legs or pelvis. Symptoms of a large embolus include sudden onset of anxiety and tachypnea. Tachycardia, palpitations, fever, or syncope may occur, and unilateral wheezing may be a prominent sign. In the elderly, angina-like pain is common. Blood gases show hypoxemia and possibly a low PCO_2. However, indolent phlebothrombosis more commonly sheds numbers of smaller emboli over a period of a few days, producing increasing cardiac and pulmonary failure without any of the localizing signs described above.

D. Sleep apnea (Ancoli-Israel & Kripke, 1986) is a disorder of multiple interruptions of respiration (more than 30 per night, each over 10 seconds) during sleep. It may result from pharyngeal obstruction, failure of central respiratory drive, or a mixture of both, is heralded by loud snoring, and is followed by disturbance of sleep (parasomnia). Its incidence increases after middle age and often is accompanied by nocturnal myoclonus, a repetitive spasm of the leg muscles. Both conditions result in a patient who seems to be always sleepy in the daytime. Impairment of cognitive function, depression, and personality changes have been linked to the disorders. Apnea is likely to produce cardiac arrhythmias, hypertension, and circulatory failure; in one laboratory series, death occurred within one year of diagnosis in 20% of those not treated. Diagnosis should be confirmed by a polysomnogram in a sleep laboratory. Treatment may include surgical correction of obstruction.

VIII. Gastrointestinal Disorders
(Chopra & Curtis, 1985)

These embrace a major area of concern of the elderly, and the ability to address the many complaints of older patients is essential to the maintenance of good communication and primary care.
  A. Acquired loss of teeth (Kamen & Sherman, 1981) affects most older people; 50% are edentulous, 25% have dentures that they do not wear, and 33% of denture wearers have lesions due to them. Prevention and treatment of periodontal disease is often the key to avoiding loss of teeth. Socioeconomic factors are critical in determining the level of care received. Psychiatric issues may include nutrition, phonation, and self-esteem.
  B. Functional digestive disorders were diagnosed in 56% of all elderly patients seen in a typical GI clinic. Complaints included pain, nausea, acid regurgitation, and cramping.
    1. Esophageal motility abnormalities (Marshall, 1985) are common in the aged. Those of particular interest to geriatric psychiatrists include:
      a. Dysphagia, which is almost never psychogenic. It may be due to neuromuscular dysfunction, such as achalasia, and then involves liquids initially. In achalasia, large amounts of food may be regurgitated and a wide dilatation of the esophagus is seen on barium swallow. Treatment is by dilatation. If the dysphagia begins with solid food, a working diagnosis of cancer is appropriate unless another organic cause of stricture can be demonstrated.
      b. Pseudobulbar palsy is seen in cerebrovascular disease and dementia. When a liquid is swallowed, some is directed into the larynx. This produces a fit of coughing, and occasionally syncope, and is followed by aspiration pneumonitis of some degree. If frequent, dehydration can result and a gastrostomy may be indicated.
      c. Presbyesophagus refers to a neuromotor abnormality seen at all ages but more common in the old, associated with diabetes, Parkinson's disease, and dementia. Metoclopropamide may be helpful in treatment.
      d. Odynophagia and esophageal spasm may resemble angina. It may respond to nitroglycerine, making a differentiation from

angina difficult. Treatment is with anticholinergics (whose side effects may be of concern in the elderly) and the avoidance of cold drinks.
   e. Hiatus hernia has a frequency of 50% at age 70 but often cannot be correlated with symptoms. Informing an asymptomatic patient of an incidental finding of a hiatus hernia may produce unnecessary anxiety. On the other hand, incorrectly ascribing to a hiatus hernia a role in the etiology of retrosternal pain may result in false reassurance and a failure to diagnose angina.
2. Gastric and duodenal abnormalities are also common causes of symptoms in older patients.
   a. Chronic atrophic gastritis is commoner as age advances; it results in achlorhydria. Antibodies to intrinsic factor develop in some cases (Type A), and this may lead to pernicious anemia. In others (Type B) dyspepsia and ulcer are common. Carcinoma is a complication of both types.
   b. Peptic ulcers (Grossman et al., 1981) occur in 10% of the elderly, and a fifth of all new ulcers begin after age 60; these result in 80% of ulcer deaths at all ages. Ulcers of the stomach and duodenum occur in equal numbers in late life. Many are associated with aspirin use, which is common in late life because of the prevalence of arthritis and of self-medication. Ironically, effervescent aspirin preparations may be taken erroneously for the relief of dyspepsia. The classical pain syndromes of postprandial or nocturnal pain are seen less commonly than atypical dyspepsia; many patients presenting with a hemorrhage have been asymptomatic. Treatment is difficult, due to the frequent complications of standard antiulcer therapy; antacids cause hypernatremia, trisilicates cause constipation, magnesia and phosphate cause osmotic diarrhea, magnesium toxicity, hypercalcemia, alumina hypophosphatemia, alkalosis, and interfere with the absorption of antibiotics; anticholinergics cause delirium; cimetidine interacts with the hepatic metabolism of some psychotherapeutic agents and frequently causes mental confusion; ranitidine causes less mental confusion; sucralfate causes constipation.
3. Colonic and rectal function is of major concern to many elderly.
   a. Constipation (Coni, Davison, & Webster, 1980) is often intolerable to older Americans who were taught to believe a daily stool is an essential of continued existence. The most frequent cause of failure to pass daily stools lies in the low-residue diet of our culture, a lack of adequate water intake,

insufficient physical exercise, and a dependency on laxatives. Inconvenience, especially in the restrained and disabled, painful anal lesions, obstruction, and debility must also be considered. Depression commonly is accompanied by constipation, which can be aggravated by the use of tricyclics. The "five constipated aunties" should be recognized readily—antidepressant, anticholinergic, antiparkinson, antacid, and analgesics (with codeine). Constipated demented patients require reminders because they cannot remember to defecate; failure may result in agitation, subsequent use of tranquilizers that may have paradoxical effects, and worsening of both the delirium and the constipation.

b. Fecal incontinence (Smith, 1983) is often reversible, for example, if caused by unrecognized fecal impaction, urgency of bowel emptying, or overuse of cathartics. Incontinence in neurologically impaired older people may be unavoidable, but regular encopresis in a demented patient can often be forestalled by the quaintly termed "bowel-training" techniques.

c. Irritable bowel syndrome (LaMont & Isselbacher, 1986) is more common in middle than in old age, but persists far into late life. Depressive, hysterical, and obsessive-compulsive personalities are predisposed to the syndrome; prevalence is twice as common in women as in men. The common pattern, known as "spastic colon," a misnomer, is typified by constipation and colicky lower abdominal pain with increased peristalsis; another symptom complex, which may occur alone or alternate with colic, has a characteristic watery diarrhea, no pain, and low peristaltic activity. Small amounts of drugs may be needed for the most severe attacks, but counseling the patient to avoid stressful situations that may trigger attacks is the best therapy. Diagnostic workup may include sigmoidoscopy, barium enema, and stool specimen for blood and parasites; the goal is to rule out inflammatory and other bowel conditions such as ulcerative colitis and Crohn's colitis, diverticulitis, and tumor. Thyrotoxicosis and lactase deficiency should also be considered. In general, the length of the history is understandably discouraging to the patient, but it is this feature that can most reassure the physician that the diagnosis is correct.

d. Diverticulosis (Johnson & Block, 1985) is an asymptomatic incidental finding on the barium enema unless it results in complications.

e. Diverticulitis is an acute febrile painful condition that may present as an acute abdomen. It is due to rupture of a diver-

ticulum and consequent localization as an abscess. Treatment is conservative except in peritonitis.
   f. Acquired megacolon is seen in individuals who have long-standing schizophrenia or depression, especially if institutionalized. It consists of a tremendously dilated, painless colon. Unlike true Hirschsprung's disease, the rectum is also loaded with feces. Patients with Parkinson's and other neurological disease, and those receiving long-term narcotics and neuroleptics, may have similar but lesser colonic retention.
   g. Lactase deficiency is seen in families of Mediterranean origin more than others. Most sufferers recognize their intolerance of milk. The elderly may be subjected to the rather common tendency of caretakers to emphasize milk products and not be in a position to object. In lactase deficiency a high milk or milk-product diet results in a colicky, osmotic diarrhea, with sour-smelling flatus, which disappears if the milk is withheld. Stools of this kind may be accepted by caregivers as part of the normal changes of aging, and the remedy of avoiding milk is then not considered.

IX. Genitourinary Disorders

A. Urinary incontinence (Coni, Davison, & Webster, 1980) may affect 20% of those over age 65, and a higher percentage of institutionalized elderly.
   1. Reversible (Gregory & Purcell, 1986) causes can be treated, but success in "toilet training" requires some degree of cooperation from the patient. Treatable causes include:
      a. Diuresis: nocturnal (incipient heart failure); diuretic (coffee, drugs); osmotic (hyperglycemia).
      b. Inflammatory: urinary tract infection; vaginitis.
      c. Mechanical: prostatic and trigonal bladder neck obstruction (retention overflow); fecal obstruction; urethral displacement (stress incontinence).
      d. Psychological: regression; personality disorder.
      e. Iatrogenic: sedation; anticholinergics; diuretics; sympathomimetics.
   2. Irreversible causes require diagnosis and counseling. It is very frustrating for a patient with neurological incontinence to be subjected to the pressures of "toilet training."
      a. Dementia: deteriorating cortical inhibition; micturition apraxia.
      b. Neurogenic: parietal; paraplegic; peripheral neuritis.
      c. Iatrogenic: post-prostatectomy complications.

3. Management is designed to diagnose and correct reversible causes and, in established cases, to channel, contain, and absorb the urine. A thorough physical examination, urinalysis and culture, an IVP with cystogram if indicated, dynamic flow studies, and cystoscopy are desirable. Counseling the patient and family is challenging because feelings of reticence, anger, and hopelessness may be encountered; it is rewarding if the quality of life is improved.

B. Benign prostatic hyperplasia (BPH) is present in 75% of males over 75. It causes a great deal of morbidity, and considerable mortality due to renal failure.
  1. Symptoms (Breschi, 1983) may be:
     a. Obstructive: that is, hesitancy; straining; decreased force and caliber; prolonged dribbling; sense of incomplete emptying; and urinary retention. Bladder hemorrhage is an indirect effect of obstruction. It is important to understand that atropine-like drugs, including many neuroleptics and tricyclics, aggravate obstructive symptoms, and drugs that relieve these symptoms (e.g., dibenzyline) may cause behavioral effects. Coffee, alcohol, and tobacco increase obstructive symptoms, as does an overdistended bladder.
     b. Irritative: that is, frequency; urgency; nocturia; dysuria. All are due to overflow incontinence, detrusor instability, urinary tract infection, or prostatitis.
     c. Neurogenic: that is, arise coincidentally to BPH. This is a relative contraindication to prostatectomy, since symptoms cannot be properly evaluated.
  2. *Examination* should ensure estimates of the size of the prostate and bladder and attempt to exclude the presence of carcinoma. Diagnostic tests may include uroflowmetry, IVP, and cysto-urethroscopy. For incontinence, cystography is included. The psychiatrist has an important role to play as consultant because of widespread doubt and fear of castration. After transurethral prostatectomy (TURP), the majority of previously potent patients continue to be potentially orgasmic; ejaculatory force is less, but potency increases as often as it is lost. However, many men date the onset of impotence to the operation; this is probably due to a lack of psychological support before and after surgery.

C. Male sexual dysfunction (Ham, 1986) due to organic causes may appear in the form of erectile and ejaculatory difficulties because of arterial insufficiency (e.g., Leriche syndrome due to iliac artery obstruction), neurological disease (e.g., autonomic neuropathy in diabetes, organic brain syndrome), drug use (Segraves, 1983) (e.g., neuroleptics, antidepressants, alphamethyldopa, cimetidine, alcohol), genitourinary disease (e.g., prostatitis, surgery), and debilitating conditions (e.g., leukemia, renal failure, fever). Many of these require involvement of the psychiatrist as therapist or consultant.

D. Gynecological disorders (Glowacki, 1983) are often neglected because of the reluctance of older women to seek examination. Many ills are due to estropenic atrophy and can be relieved by local therapy. There is much controversy regarding systemic estrogens in women over 60. Minor vulval and vaginal abnormalities are common; they cause discomfort and a disproportionate amount of worry. Thorough histories should include specific inquiries about physical symptoms and sexual functioning.

X. Failure of Temperature Regulation (Besdine & Harris, 1985)

A. Accidental hypothermia may occur in the mentally impaired, alcoholic, or chronically ill elderly and has a high mortality. Etiologically, immobility, endocrine disorders, starvation, neuroleptics, sedatives, and CVA have all been implicated. Living in a cool room may be enough to cause hypothermia of gradual onset, which may be difficult to distinguish from dementia or lacunar stroke. All elderly admissions to hospitals in cool seasons should have the initial rectal temperature recorded by an electronic instrument, since glass thermometers do not show low readings. As body temperature decreases, shivering ceases (32°C) and impaired consciousness occurs, reducing the instinct for self-preservation; bradycardia, low blood pressure, and slow respirations follow. Below that, atrial fibrillation occurs (30°C), then ventricular fibrillation. Rewarming techniques are controversial, but to avoid lethal metabolic complications slow spontaneous rewarming in a postoperative recovery room is preferred over heating.

B. Hyperthermia occurs when body temperature is above 41°C; over 41.5°C death is frequent. Heat cramps and heat exhaustion are usually seen in younger individuals and are readily reversible; heat stroke or hyperpyrexia is an overwhelming dysfunction of temperature regulation, and 80% of the mortality from it is reported in those over age 50. Anhidrosis and severe CNS disturbances occur. Etiological risk factors include infection, burns, intracranial conditions (including trauma, hemorrhage, tumor, and inflammation), alcoholic withdrawal, and drugs. Postanesthetic malignant pyrexia and malignant neuroleptic syndrome appear to be variants of hyperthermia. Iatrogenically induced syndromes have in common the administration of atropine cogeners (antiparkinson medication, tricyclic antidepressants, and certain neuroleptics), all of which appear to impair the ability to regulate temperature. There has been some controversy about which neuroleptics are most responsible, and haloperidol is suspected of having a special liability. However, it appears that all have this potential; the high number of initial reports of haloperidol hyperpyrexia reflects the heavy usage of the drug and the heightened sensitivity to the supposed relationship created by reports.

XI. Diseases of the Joints and Connective Tissue (Calkins, Papademetriou, & Challa, 1986)

These are the basis of numerous common complaints in the elderly. In most health surveys, over 50% of respondents over age 65 report significant symptoms relating to bones and connective tissue.

A. Metabolic joint disease is summarized in the section on metabolic disease.
B. Degenerative joint disease, or osteoarthritis, has two forms: (1) local, or posttraumatic, and (2) generalized, affecting progressively the hands, knees, hips and spine.
  1. Diagnosis usually follows physical examination, prompted either by symptoms or an incidental observation. Confirmation is by x-ray, since radiological changes are present before symptoms, in contrast to inflammatory arthritis. Treatment utilizes physical measures to relieve pain and spasm, analgesics and other drugs, both orally and by injection into the joint, and prosthetic surgery. Treatment and rehabilitation offer many opportunities for the geropsychiatrist to become a significant member of a team. Studies of the role of stress in precipitating attacks and injuries, the psychology of motivation in rehabilitation, and treatment of concomitant depression are examples of psychiatric tasks.
C. Rheumatoid arthritis has a peak incidence in late maturity but highest prevalence in old age. Many patients enter late life with a legacy of deformity, but in other patients the disease begins after age 60; about 75% of the latter have a subacute mild course without many systemic manifestations, and although pain does not always respond to analgesics it can be readily controlled by low-dose steroids; the prognosis for remission in subacute arthritis is, however, rather poor. The minority of patients have an acute explosive illness, but clinical remission is common in this acute form of the illness.

D. Polymyalgia rheumatica (PMR) is a disease almost exclusively seen in the aged. After a period of low-grade fever and weight loss, polymyalgia develops in the musculature of the pectoral girdle and to a lesser extent around the hips. Depression is very frequent, and some patients become frankly paranoid. Blood examination shows an impressive rise of the sedimentation rate, mild anemia, with a normal white count and absent rheumatoid factor. Steroid therapy is effective for both the connective tissue disease and the psychiatric symptoms. Nonsteroidal anti-inflammatory drugs can also be used.
E. Giant cell arteritis has a strong familial incidence and mostly affects whites. The onset is insidious, with fever malaise and weight loss, occasionally with confusional syndrome or depression. Diagnosis and control of symptoms with high-dose steriods should be considered medical emergencies because in the 25-50% of cases with ocular involvement there is the potential of sudden blindness.
F. Gout and pseudogout are common causes of acute arthritis in the elderly. Gout should be suspected if the serum uric acid is above 9mg./dl, but is not confirmed unless uric acid crystals are seen in a joint aspirate. Pseudogout is a similar acute arthritis due to precipitation of calcium pyrophosphate crystals. Synovial fluid for culture and microscopic examination should be drawn from all acutely inflamed joints to rule out septic arthritis. Acute flareup of rheumatoid, lupus, or psoriatic arthritis should also be considered. Treatment includes nonsteroidal anti-inflammatory drugs, all of which can cause confusional symptoms in the elderly.
G. Paget's disease (Wallach, 1985) of bone occurs in 1-3% of the population over 50 years of age. It is associated with intranuclear inclusion bodies, in some cases suggesting a "slow virus" etiology. Most cases are asymptomatic, having been discovered because of a casual reading of a high alkaline phosphatase or an incidental finding in an x-ray. New drugs are very useful and might be expected to reduce the complications experienced by a minority. Whether the incidence of bone sarcoma will be reduced by treatment remains to be seen.

XII. Summary

A thorough knowledge of internal medicine is immeasurably beneficial for the practicing geropsychiatrist. There are many aspects of internal medicine that enter into the diagnosis and care of the elderly patient. The importance of differentiation of psychiatric syndromes from those seen by other physician specialists is illustrated by the symptoms of depression and myxedema. Recognizing the organic basis of psychiatric symptoms is important in the workup of delirium. Knowing about the limitations imposed by physical disease upon proposed psychiatric treatment is important in, for example, using tricyclics where cardiac conduction disorders exist, or where there would be interference between drug therapies, such as occurs with the depressed patient with COPD. With the growth of interdisciplinary treatment teams, the role of the psychiatrist has become less isolated and psychiatric contributions more sought after. There is a need for someone who can see the patient as a whole, just as the patient sees himself or herself. This "primary therapist" or holistic role may fall to the psychiatrist by plan or default. In such circumstances there is a need to be familiar with the internist's approach to disease (Rowe, 1985). Fortunately, the psychiatrist is already quite familiar with this view of general medicine; much of the material in this chapter will be remembered from years of training in medical school, residency, and clinical practice; use of the bibliography and current update articles (Rosenthal, 1985) should establish this as a continuous process.

REFERENCES

American Cancer Society Task Force on Breast Cancer Control. (1982). *Statement on mammography. Ca. 32*, 226–230.
Ancoli-Israel, S., & Kripke, D. F. (1986). Sleep and aging. In E. Calkins, P. J. Davis, & A. B. Ford (Eds.), *Practice of geriatrics* (pp. 240–247). Philadelphia: Saunders.
Applegate, W. B. (1986). Systolic hypertension: When and how to treat. In R. J. Ham (Ed.), *Geriatric medicine annual* (pp. 40–54). Oradell, NJ: Medical Economics.
Barber, H. R. K. (1986). Ovarian cancer. *Ca. 36*, 149–184.
Bartlett, J. G. (1985). Pneumonia. In R. Andres, E. L. Bierman, & W. R. Hazzard (Eds.), *Principles of geriatric medicine* (pp. 554–562). New York: McGraw-Hill.
Barzel, U. (1983). Vitamin D deficiency: A risk factor for osteomalacia in the aged. *J Amer Geriat Soc, 31*, 598–601.
Besdine, R. W., & Harris, T. B. (1985). Alterations in the body temperature: Hypothermia and hyperthermia. In R. Andres, E. L. Bierman, & W. R. Hazzard (Eds.), *Principles of geriatric medicine* (pp. 209–217). New York: McGraw-Hill.
Brendler, C. B. (1985). Disorders of the prostate. In R. Andres, E. L. Bierman, & W. R. Hazzard (Eds.), *Principles of geriatric medicine* (pp. 647–652). New York: McGraw-Hill.
Breschi, L. (1983). Common lower urinary tract problems in the elderly. In W. Reichel (Ed.), *Clinical aspects of aging* (pp. 302–319). Baltimore: Williams & Wilkins.

Brown, R., & Scharf, S. M. (1985). Pulmonary embolism and chronic obstructive pulmonary disease. In T. M. Walshe (Ed.), *Manual of clinical problems in geriatric medicine* (pp. 210-215). Boston: Little, Brown.

Cahill, G. F. (1983). Hyperglycemic hyperosmolar coma: A syndrome almost unique to the elderly. *J Amer Geriat Soc, 31*, 103-105.

Caird, F. I. (1982). Valvular disease of the heart. In D. Platt (Ed.), *Geriatrics I* (pp. 93-108). New York: Springer-Verlag.

Calkins, E., Papademetriou, T., & Challa, H. R. (1986). Musculoskeletal diseases in the elderly. In E. Calkins, P. J. Davis, & A. B. Ford (Eds.), *Practice of geriatrics* (pp. 386-430). Philadelphia: Saunders.

Chiodo, G. T., Eigner, T., & Rosenstein, D. I. (1986). Oral cancer detection. *Postgrad Med, 80*, 231-236.

Chopra, S., & Curtis, R. L. (1985). Gastrointestinal diseases. In T. M. Walshe (Ed.), *Manual of clinical problems in geriatric medicine* (pp. 183-206). Boston: Little, Brown.

Clamon, G. H., Audeh, M. W., & Pinnick, S. (1982). Small cell lung carcinoma in the elderly. *J Amer Geriat Soc, 30*, 299-302.

Coni, N., Davison, W., & Webster, S. (1980). *Lecture notes on geriatrics*. Oxford: Blackwell.

Crantz, J. G. (1985). Vitamin B_{12} deficiency in the elderly. *Clinics in Geriat Med, 1*(4), 701-710.

Davis, P. J., & Davis, F. B. (1983). Endocrinology and aging. In W. Reichel (Ed.), *Clinical aspects of aging* (pp. 396-411). Baltimore: Williams & Wilkins.

Delmez, J. A. (1983). Fluid and electrolyte disturbances. In J. W. Campbell & M. Frisse (Eds.), *Manual of medical therapeutics* (24th ed.) (pp. 23-43). Boston: Little, Brown.

Eddy, D. (1980). Guidelines for the cancer-related checkup: Recommendations and rationale. *Ca, 30*, 194-240.

Esposito, A. L., Gleckman, R. A., & Cram, S. (1980). Community-acquired bacteremia in the elderly. *J Amer Geriat Soc, 28*, 315-316.

Evans, D. L., Edelson, G. A., & Golden, R. N. (1983). Organic psychosis without anemia or spinal cord symptoms in patients with vitamin B_{12} deficiency. *Amer J Psychiatry, 140*, 218.

Fleg, J. L., & Kennedy, H. L. (1982). Cardiac arrhythmias in a healthy geriatric population. *Chest, 81*, 302-307.

Foley, C. J., Libow, L. S., & Sherman, F. (1981). Clinical aspects of nutrition. In L. S. Libow & F. T. Sherman (Eds.), *The core of geriatric medicine* (pp. 280-305). St. Louis: Mosby.

Foley, K. M. (1986). The treatment of pain in the patient with cancer. *Ca, 36*, 194-215.

Frocht, A., & Fillit, H. (1984). Renal disease and the geriatric patient. *J Amer Geriat Soc, 32*, 28-43.

Gandhavadi, B., Rosen, J. S., & Addison, R. G. (1982). Autonomic pain. *Postgrad Med, 71*, 85-90.

Gilbert, P. L. (1986). Thyroid disease in the elderly. In R. J. Ham (Ed.), *Geriatric medicine annual* (pp. 213-237). Oradell, NJ: Medical Economics.

Gleckman, R. A., & Ganz, N. M. (1983). *Infections in the elderly*. Boston: Little, Brown.
Glowacki, G. (1983). Geriatric gynecology. In W. Reichel (Ed.), *Clinical aspects of aging* (pp. 319-328). Baltimore: Williams & Wilkins.
Goldberg, A. P., Andres, R., & Bierman, E. L. (1985). Diabetes in the elderly. In R. Andres, E. L. Bierman, & W. R. Hazzard (Eds.), *Principles of geriatric medicine* (pp. 750-763). New York: McGraw-Hill.
Gordon, M., & Hurowitz, E. (1984). Cardiopulmonary resuscitation in the elderly. *J Amer Geriat Soc, 32*, 930-934.
Gregory, J. G., & Purcell, M. H. (1986). Urinary incontinence in the elderly: Ways to relieve it without surgery. *Postgrad Med, 80*, 253-262.
Grinblat, J. (1985). Folate status in the aged. *Clinics in Geriat Med, 1*(4), 711-728.
Grossman, M. I., Kurata, J. H., Rotter, J. I., Meyer, J. H., Robert, A., Richardson, C. T., Debas, J. T., & Jensen, D. N. (1981). Peptic ulcer: New therapies, new diseases. *Ann Intern Med, 95*, 609-627.
Hale, Stewart, R. B., & Marks, R. G. (1984). Central nervous symptoms of elderly subjects using hypertensive drugs. *J Amer Geriat Soc, 32*, 5.
Ham, R. J. (1986). Sexual dysfunction in the elderly. In R. J. Ham (Ed.), *Geriatric medicine annual* (pp. 248-259). Oradell, NJ: Medical Economics.
Harnisch, J. P. (1984). Zoster in the elderly. *J Amer Geriat Soc, 32*, 789-793.
Harris, R. Cardiac arrhythmias. In D. Platt (Ed.), *Geriatrics I* (pp. 109-138). New York: Springer-Verlag.
Holmes, K. K. (1983). Syphilis. In R. G. Petersdorf, R. D. Adams, E. Braunwald, K. J. Isselbacher, J. B. Martin, & J. D. Wilson (Eds.), *Harrison's principles of internal medicine* (10th ed.) (pp. 1034-1045). New York: McGraw-Hill.
Johnson, H. C. L., & Block, M. A. (1985). Diverticular disease. *Postgrad Med, 78*, 75-82.
Kamen, S., & Sherman, F. T. (1981). Oral and dental disorders. In L. S. Libow & F. T. Sherman (Eds.), *The core of geriatric medicine* (pp. 305-329). St. Louis: Mosby.
Katz, R. J. (1986). New treatment methods in cardiology: Angina, CHF and arrhythmias. In R. J. Ham (Ed.), *Geriatric medicine annual* (pp. 185-197). Oradell, NJ: Medical Economics.
Klein, I., & Levey, G. S. (1984). Unusual manifestations of hypothyroidism. *Arch Int Med, 144*, 123.
Kleinfeld, M., Peter, S., & Gilbert, G. M. (1984). Delirium as the predominant manifestation of hyperparathyroidism: Reversal after parathyroidectomy. *J Amer Geriat Soc, 32*, 689-690.
Kotler, M. N., Mintz, G. S., Parry, W. R., & Segal, B. L. (1981). Bedside diagnosis of organic murmurs in the elderly. *Geriatrics, 36*, 107-125.
Lafferty, F. W. (1981). Primary hyperparathyroidism. *Arch Int Med, 141*, 1761-1766.
LaMont, J. T., & Isselbacher, K. J. (1986). Irritable bowel syndrome. In R. G. Petersdorf, R. D. Adams, E. Braunwald, K. J. Isselbacher, J. B. Martin, & J. D. Wilson (Eds.), *Harrison's principles of internal medicine* (12th ed.) (pp. 1757-1758). New York: McGraw-Hill.

Lawrence, W., Jr. (1986). Gastric cancer. *Ca, 36,* 216–236.
Lindenfeld, J., & Groves, B. M. (1982). Cardiovascular function and disease in the aged. In S. A. Schrier (Ed.), *Clinical internal medicine in the aged* (pp. 87–113). Philadelphia: Saunders.
Marshall, J. B. (1985). Dysphagia: Pathophysiology, causes and evaluation. *Postgrad Med, 77,* 58–68.
Moe, R. E. (1985). Breast diseases of elderly women. In R. Andres, E. L. Bierman, & W. R. Hazzard (Eds.), *Principles of geriatric medicine* (pp. 636–646). New York: McGraw-Hill.
Moss, A. J. (1986). Cardiac disorders somewhat specific to the elderly: Clinical syndromes, diagnostic studies and cardiac therapeutics. In E. Calkins, P. J. Davis, & A. B. Ford (Eds.), *Practice of geriatrics* (pp. 310–326). Philadelphia: Saunders.
Nelson, J. H., Averette, H. E., & Richart, R. M. (1984). Dysplasia, carcinoma in situ, and early invasive cervical carcinoma. *Ca, 34,* 306–327.
Peterson, B. A., & Kennedy, B. J. (1979). Aging and cancer management. *Ca, 29,* 322–332.
Peterson, L. G., & Perl, M. (1982, June). Psychiatric symptoms in cancer. *Psychosomatics.*
Raisz, L. G. (1982). Osteoporosis. *J Amer Geriat Soc, 30,* 127–138.
Robbins, N., de Maria, A., & Miller, M. H. (1980). Infective endocarditis in the elderly. *Southern Med J, 73,* 1335–1338.
Robinson, J. K., & Roenigk, H. H., Jr. (1980). The big three of skin cancer: Basal cell carcinoma, squamous cell carcinoma, and malignant melanoma. *Postgrad Med, 67,* 92–97.
Rodstein, M. (1971). Heart disease in the aged. In I. Rossman (Ed.), *Clinical geriatrics* (pp. 143–163). Philadelphia: Lippincott.
Rosenthal, M. (1985). Geriatrics: A selected up-to-date bibliography. *J Amer Geriat Soc, 33,* 69–85.
Rowe, J. W. (1985). Health care of the elderly. *New England J Med, 312,* 827–835.
Salcman, M. (1982). Brain tumors and the geriatric patient. *J Amer Geriat Soc, 30,* 501–508.
Santinga, J. T., Flora, J., Kirsch, M., & Baublis, J. (1983). Aortic valve replacement in the elderly. *J Amer Geriat Soc, 31,* 211–212.
Scheibel, W., & Raczek, J. (1985). Herpes simplex encephalitis. *J Fam Pract, 20,* 23–32.
Segraves, R. T. (1983). Male sexual dysfunction and psychoactive drug use. *J Amer Geriat Soc, 31,* 227–233.
Seligman, P. A. (1982). Hematological problems in the elderly. In S. A. Schrier (Ed.), *Clinical internal medicine in the aged* (pp. 280–295). Philadelphia: Saunders.
Shands, J. W. (1979). What is the role of vaccines in treating the older patient? *Geriatrics, 34,* 62–65.
Silber, R. (1982). Chronic lymphatic leukemia in the elderly. *Hosp Practice, 17,* 131.
Slovic, D. M. (1985). Carbohydrate metabolism and complications of diabetes. In T. M. Walshe (Ed.), *Manual of clinical problems in geriatric medicine* (pp. 139–146). Boston: Little, Brown.

Smith, I. M. (1986). Septicemia and bacterial endocarditis in the elderly. In E. Calkins, P. J. Davis, & A. B. Ford (Eds.), *Practice of geriatrics* (pp. 549–553). Philadelphia: Saunders.

Smith, R. G. (1983). Fecal incontinence. *J Amer Geriat Soc, 31,* 694–698.

Snyder, D. W. (1985). Mitral valve prolapse. *Postgrad Med, 77,* 281–288.

Stead, W. W., & Dutt, A. K. (1985). The changing picture in tuberculosis. In R. Andres, E. L. Bierman, & W. R. Hazzard (Eds.), *Principles of geriatric medicine* (pp. 562–571). New York: McGraw-Hill.

Stroehlein, J. R., Goulston, K., & Hunt, R. H. (1984). Diagnostic approach to evaluating the cause of a positive fecal occult blood test. *Ca, 34,* 148–157.

Stults, B. M. (1982). Digoxin use in the elderly. *J Amer Geriat Soc, 30,* 158–164.

Sutherland, A. M. (1956). Psychological impact of cancer and its therapy. *Med Clin North Amer, 40,* 705–720.

Thompson, A. R. (1985). Disorders of hemostasis, thrombosis and antithrombotic therapy. In R. Andres, E. L. Bierman, & W. R. Hazzard (Eds.), *Principles of geriatric medicine* (pp. 709–727). New York: McGraw-Hill.

Wallach, S. (1985). Paget's disease of bone. In E. Calkins, P. J. Davis, & A. B. Ford (Eds.), *Practice of geriatrics* (pp. 431–440). Philadelphia: Saunders.

Walshe, T. M. (1985). Transient neurological symptoms and signs; Thrombotic strokes; Lacunar strokes; Embolic strokes. In T. M. Walshe (Ed.), *Manual of clinical problems in geriatric medicine* (pp. 330–342). Boston: Little, Brown.

5
Principles of Diagnosis and Treatment in Geriatric Psychiatry

James E. Spar

I. Introduction

There are several modifications of traditional psychiatric diagnosis and treatment that are especially useful with the elderly. Information from several informants may be necessary, since details of past experiences may be less well recalled by the older patient. Past and present medical and surgical conditions and their treatments may clarify current psychiatric signs and symptoms. Active interview techniques (including sitting close, speaking more loudly and slowly, and allowing ample time for responses) are often useful. Attention is paid to culturally derived attitudes toward symptoms and their expression, as well as precepts regarding self-reliance, independence, and attitudes toward psychiatry and psychiatrists. In the interpretation of mental-status examination findings, allowance is made for the effects of age, chronic medical conditions and their treatments, and sociocultural factors.

Treatment of elderly patients proceeds with due attention to age-related changes in perception (e.g., vision and hearing) and drug pharmacokinetics and pharmacodynamics. Some elderly patients respond especially to the therapist's expressions of concern; thus "symbolic giving" (e.g., offering a cup of tea) and physical expressions of affection and concern (e.g., a pat on the shoulder) may be especially well received by the elderly.

Perhaps most importantly, the psychiatrist avoids therapeutic pessimism and nihilism. Even though the elderly patient is in closer proximity to death, the physician tries to utilize modern therapeutic strategies to achieve realistic goals.

Principles of patient management sometimes require modification with elderly patients. Transportation difficulties may call for more extensive use of telephone contact. The psychiatrist may need to function in different roles because of rapid changes in the patient's condition. For example, the psychiatrist may function as a case coordinator—necessitating contact with other professionals, family members, and neighbors—or, at other times, as a family therapist. Finally, indications for psychiatric hospitalization are sometimes broader for the elderly patient, with deteriorating self-care and coexisting medical conditions serving as indications for hospitalization along with the more traditional categories of danger to self or others and psychosis.

II. Goals of Psychiatric Assessment and Treatment (Comfort, 1980; Verwoerdt, 1976)

A. Primary goals—psychiatric treatment of the elderly patient pursues three parallel goals: amelioration of symptoms, restoration of functioning, and enhancement of subjective quality of life.
   1. Amelioration of symptoms: In this context, symptom is taken to mean both those sensations recorded by patient complaints (classical symptoms) and those features of illness observed by the physician (classical signs). Although patients and physicians may not agree on what are truly symptoms (as opposed to abnormal awareness of, or reaction to, normal sensations), the physician treating elderly patients, in general, regards all patient complaints as proper targets for inquiry and intervention. As evaluation and treatment progress, both patient and physician may agree to redefine treatment goals in terms of a modified cluster of symptoms. At times, the goal of achieving total eradication of symptoms may seriously impair attainment of the other goals discussed below, in which case it may be appropriate to allow some symptoms to remain incompletely resolved.
   2. Restoration of optimal functioning: This treatment goal requires the physician to identify appropriate norms of function, taking into account the patient's premorbid functional level as well as the limitations imposed by advanced age, physical illness, and the opportunities currently afforded by the patient's physical and social environment. Assessment is made of various functional levels: physiological, psychomotor, intrapsychic, interpersonal,

social, and occupational. At times, establishment of appropriate norms for all of these levels of functioning may comprise the greater part of the overall diagnostic effort, particularly in patients with chronic and/or deteriorating conditions. Often, intervention is directed toward family members as well as the identified elderly patient, even though the relationship between the identified elderly patient and the physician remains the first priority. In other cases, the intervention may be directed toward the patient's physical environment in an attempt to compensate for age- and disease-related reduction of physical and emotional capacities.
   3. Enhancement of the subjective quality of life: The physician encourages the patient to realistically appraise and utilize his or her remaining strengths and environmental resources to compensate for some of the biopsychosocial losses associated with aging. Treatment encourages the patient to enjoy remaining pleasures in life (e.g., grandchildren, retirement, intellectual curiosity) and to maintain as much independence, self-esteem, and dignity as is possible. With some elderly patients, goals may include heightened insight and self-awareness, comfort in accepting one's mortality and unrealized aspirations, and comfort in one's religious beliefs.

III. Technical Considerations
(Butler & Lewis, 1982; Jarvik & Small, 1982; Miller, 1977)

A. The psychiatrist employs all of the techniques of modern medicine and general psychiatry to achieve realistic goals for each patient. Available modalities include:
   1. The medical and psychiatric history supplemented, when indicated, by interviews of family and friends.
   2. The physical and neurological examination (including assessment of visual and auditory acuity).
   3. The comprehensive mental-status examination (supplemented by appropriate psychological and neuropsychological tests); laboratory tests; consultation with other medical and nonmedical specialists; and inpatient, day hospital, and outpatient treatment, including administration of pharmacologic, psychotherapeutic (including conjoint, group, and family therapy), and electroconvulsive therapy.
B. Specific techniques for elderly patients include:
   1. The therapist's adoption of an optimistic stance.
   2. Use of active engagement (as opposed to more passive listening).

3. The employment of symbolic and real giving.
4. Physical expressions of concern.
C. Other modifications take into account sensory and cognitive impairments. These include:
1. Sitting close.
2. Speaking loudly and slowly with frequent repetition.
3. Use of sound-amplifying devices.
4. Provision of ample time for responses.

IV. The History
(Comfort, 1980; Verwoerdt, 1976)

A. The present illness includes:
1. The temporal sequence of symptom development.
2. The relationship of symptoms to daily activities.
3. Recent life events and stresses.
4. Medication usage, including over-the-counter medications.
5. Repeated inquiries about mood and affect, since denial, repression, and suppression of affect seem to be particularly common among elderly patients.
6. Consideration of cultural and personal idiosyncracies regarding the language used by elderly patients to describe their symptoms.
7. Current treatments for concomitant medical illnesses are elicited, with particular attention to the interaction between preexisting medical conditions and the psychiatric symptoms of the present illness, as well as the interaction between medication side effects and psychiatric symptoms.
B. Compared with adult patients, greater reliance is usually placed on information from reliable informants and more time is required to obtain the necessary information. Inquiry includes:
1. A comprehensive identification of past subclinical and clinical episodes of:
   a. Affective disorder.
   b. Paranoid ideas.
   c. Cognitive dysfunction.
   d. Psychosis.
   e. Substance abuse and/or dependency.
2. Explored also are the patient's:
   a. Interpersonal relationships.
   b. Educational and intellectual development.
   c. Level of social and occupational functioning.
   d. Adaptive and maladaptive behavior during and following stressful events.

e. Use or avoidance of medical services and compliance with past treatment regimens.
  3. Early life and developmental data are covered, with particular attention to oedipal and pre-oedipal issues that may influence transference reactions to the therapist and compliance with treatment.
  4. Present cultural beliefs, expectations, and attitudes in general and, in particular, toward symptom formation, illness, and medical treatment.
  5. Precepts concerning self-reliance, dependency, and complaint behavior are important, as are past and present sexual attitudes and experiences, as well as attitudes and expectations regarding psychiatry and psychotherapy.
C. The past medical history includes:
  1. Details of past illnesses, hospitalizations, treatments, trauma, and surgeries.
  2. Particular emphasis is placed on common medical problems in the elderly that can contribute to, or present as, psychiatric signs and symptoms, such as:
     a. Hypertension.
     b. Endocrine disorders (e.g., hypothyroidism).
     c. Alterations in neurologic function (e.g., transient ischemic attacks, strokes).
     d. Cardiac function (e.g., arrythmias, infarcts, heart block).
     e. Gastrointestinal functions (e.g., previous hepatitis, malabsorption, bowel irregularities).
     f. Genitourinary functions (e.g., incontinence, hesitancy, urgency).
  3. The patient's customary dietary patterns (e.g., nutritional status, diets, special likes and dislikes, cultural or religious limitations) are explored, including use or misuse of:
     a. Vitamins.
     b. Minerals.
     c. Folk remedies.
     d. Over-the-counter medications.
     e. Food supplements.
     f. Tobacco.
     g. Alcohol.
     h. Common drugs (prescription and otherwise).
     i. Drugs of abuse (e.g., minor tranquilizers and barbiturates).
  4. Unusual changes in weight may point to depression or cognitive dysfunction.

D. Family history includes:
   1. General health status of:
      a. Parents.
      b. Siblings.
      c. Children.
      d. Grandchildren.
   2. Specific inquiry regarding the occurrence in family members of:
      a. Affective disorders.
      b. Suicide attempts and completions.
      c. Schizophrenia.
      d. Alcohol and drug abuse.
      e. Sociopathy.
      f. Age of onset and course of cognitive decline; such inquiry may also uncover a family member's apprehension about genetic predisposition to the elderly family member's dementia.

V. Mental-Status Examination
(Folstein, Folstein, & McHugh, 1975; Raskin & Jarvik, 1979; Reisberg, Ferris, de Leon, & Crook, 1982; Strub & Black, 1977)

A. Includes assessment of:
   1. General psychiatric status.
   2. Detailed assessment of cognitive functioning.
B. The use of standardized assessment instruments and rating scales is recommended, such as the following:
   1. Mini-Mental State.
   2. Inventory of Psychic and Somatic Complaints–Elderly.
   3. Beck Depression Inventory.
   4. Global Deterioration Scale.
   5. Many other available measures.
C. It is generally useful to become familiar with two or three scales that tap different functions, such as cognition, mood, and activities of daily living, and to use these scales exclusively. In this way the clinician can become experienced using these scales with a wide variety of patients and develop skill in their administration and interpretation.

VI. The Physical Examination

A. May be performed by a medical colleague or by the treating psychiatrist, depending on the clinical setting and the anticipated therapist–patient relationship. It includes:

1. A complete general physical and neurological examination, including:
   a. Measurement of orthostatic change in blood pressure.
      (1) After the patient is in a supine position for at least three minutes, blood pressure and heart rate are recorded; then the patient sits or stands up and, after two minutes, the blood pressure is again measured.
   b. Baseline measurement for orthostatic hypotension is useful for monitoring blood pressure during psychotropic drug treatment and for selecting an appropriate psychotropic medication (e.g., a high, rather than a low, potency neuroleptic may be selected for a psychotic patient who has a tendency toward orthostasis).

VII. Laboratory Evaluation
(Raskind, Peskind, Rivaro, Veith, & Barnes, 1982)

A. To uncover a medical etiology or contributing factor for the problems listed below; this list is not intended to be all-inclusive.
   1. Affective disorder.
      a. Complete blood count.
      b. Urinalysis.
      c. TSH.
      d. T_4.
      e. Electrocardiogram.
      f. SMA 18.
      g. Chest x-ray.
   2. Cognitive impairment. Above tests plus:
      a. Sedimentation rate.
      b. Vitamin B_{12}, folate.
      c. Bilirubin.
      d. VDRL or STS.
      e. Urine or blood for heavy metals if intoxication is suspected.
      f. Computer-assisted tomogram of brain.
      f. Drug screen for drugs of abuse.
   3. Specialized tests, such as:
      a. Dexamethasone suppression test (DST).
      b. Thyrotropin releasing hormone test (TRH).
   These two biological tests do not appear useful for the diagnosis of depression in this age group due to the relatively high rate of false positive and negative results associated with:
      a. Medical illnesses.

b. Appreciable weight loss.
c. Medications.
d. Dementia.
e. Endocrine disorders.

VIII. The Diagnostic Process
(American Psychiatric Association, DSM-III-R, 1987)

A. Establishing a diagnosis on all axes of the *Diagnostic and Statistical Manual-III-R* is preferable in order to consider all relevant diagnostic and treatment factors.
   1. If the dementia syndrome is identified, it is important to clarify the likely etiology and to identify contributing factors (such as depression) that may be amenable to therapeutic intervention.
   2. Recognition of the patient's predominant personality characteristics is also useful, since these traits may influence the presentation of illness, the therapeutic relationship, and treatment compliance.
   3. A record of the patient's functional level (e.g., activities of daily living), living circumstances, chronic and acute medical illnesses, and ongoing therapies can serve as a baseline against which the effects of treatment can be evaluated.
   4. Information from informants familiar with the patient's premorbid functioning is especially useful as a guide for setting treatment goals.

IX. Treatment
(Butler & Lewis, 1982; Pfeiffer, 1976; Spar, 1985; Wheatley, 1982)

A. The therapeutic relationship is the cornerstone of therapy and should be facilitated by regular office visits supplemented when necessary by phone contacts. Some elderly patients require continual contact with the psychiatrist over a lengthy period of time. Gestures of the psychiatrist's concern (e.g., a call to remind the patient of the next appointment) can strengthen the therapeutic relationship.
B. Psychoactive drug therapy is initiated with consideration of:
   1. Age-related pharmacokinetic factors.
   2. Concomitant diseases.
   3. Other medications.
      a. In general, dosages are low (one-third to one-fourth of the usual adult starting dose) and gradually raised, depending on therapeutic response and development of side effects.

C. Appropriate target symptoms are identified and reasonable periods of treatment are provided before changing treatment strategies. For example,
   1. Some elderly patients require three to five weeks before responding to an antidepressant but may enjoy improved sleep and appetite within one week of treatment.
D. Patients and responsible family members are apprised of side effects and adverse reactions and instructed to report their occurrence.
E. Appropriate adjustment of nonpsychotropic medications, as indicated, is performed in collaboration with other treating physicians. For example, the dose of an antihypertensive may need to be lowered when an antidepressant or neuroleptic that decreases blood pressure is used.
F. Elderly patients with the following problems should be considered for acute hospital care:
   1. Suicidal impulses or plans.
      a. These may or may not be verbalized by the patient.
      b. Careful assessment of verbal and nonverbal clues is important, as is supplemental information from others.
   2. Psychotic symptoms, such as hallucinations or delusions, often accompanied by behavior disturbances. These symptoms may be denied; again, other sources of information are important.
   3. Regressive behavior; for example, an elderly patient with a major psychiatric disorder who is unable to perform simple activities of daily living and unable to comply with medical and psychiatric treatment.
   4. Excessive risk to patient if treatment is administered at a less intensive level, such as:
      a. Cardiac or other medical conditions rendering pharmacologic treatment of depression too risky.
      b. Unavailability of family members to assist in monitoring and/or supervising treatment.
      c. Dementia with a depressive component being too complex for an adequate diagnostic workup to be carried out in an outpatient setting.
G. Outpatient Care.
   1. Principles are generally the same as for younger patients, except that visits for certain patients may be of shorter duration (e.g., for medication reassessment).
   2. A more active and engaging rather than a passive therapeutic role is usually appropriate.
   3. "Reminder calls" before visits may be necessary.

X. Summary

A. Psychiatric evaluation and treatment of elderly patients is similar in many ways to that provided to younger adults. Modifications especially applicable to the elderly include:
   1. Greater emphasis on assessing concomitant medical conditions.
   2. Greater use of ancillary sources of information.
   3. Adoption of a more active and optimistic attitude.
   4. Provision of more frequent visits to monitor side effects and response to treatment.
B. Psychopharmacotherapy generally employs smaller dosages and may more commonly require acute hospital admission for their safe administration.

REFERENCES

American Psychiatric Association. (1987). *Diagnostic and Statistical Manual of Mental Disorders* (3rd ed., Revised). Washington, D.C.: American Psychiatric Press.

Butler, R. N., & Lewis, M. I. (1982). General treatment principles. In D. L. Bowen (Ed.), *Aging and mental health: Positive psychosocial and biomedical approaches* (3rd ed.) (pp. 171–195). St. Louis, MO: Mosby.

Comfort, A. (1980). *Practice of geriatric psychiatry.* New York: Elsevier.

Folstein, M. F., Folstein, S. E., & McHugh, P. R. (1975). Mini-Mental State: A practical method for grading the cognitive state of patients for the clinician. *J Psychiatr Res, 12*:189–198.

Jarvik, L. F., & Small, G. W. (Eds.) (1982). *The psychiatric clinics of North America* (Vol. 5, No. 1, Aging). Philadelphia: Saunders.

Miller, E. (1977). *Abnormal aging.* New York: Wiley.

Pfeiffer, E. (1976). Psychotherapy with elderly patients. In L. Bellak & T. B. Karasu (Eds.), *Geriatric psychiatry: A handbook for psychiatrists and primary care physicians* (pp. 191–205). New York: Grune & Stratton.

Raskin, A., & Jarvik, L. F. (1979). *Psychiatric symptoms and cognitive loss in the elderly: Evaluation and assessment techniques.* Washington, DC: Hemisphere Publishing.

Raskind, M., Peskind, E., Rivaro, M. F., Veith, R., & Barnes, R. (1982). Dexamethasone suppression test and cortisol circadian rhythm in primary degenerative dementia. *Amer J Psychiat, 139,* 1468–1471.

Reisberg, B., Ferris, S. H., de Leon, M. J., & Crook, T. (1982). The global deterioration scale for assessment of primary degenerative dementia. *Am J psychiatry, 139*(9), 1136–1139.

Spar, J. (1985). Psychopharmacologic treatment of depression in elderly patients with cardiovascular disease. In C. Shamoian (Ed.), *Treatment of affective disorders in the elderly.* Washington, DC: American Psychiatric Press.

Strub, R. L., & Black, F. W. (1977). *The mental status examination in neurology.* Philadelphia: Davis.
Verwoerdt, A. (1976). *Clinical geropsychiatry.* Baltimore: Williams & Wilkins.
Wheatley, D. (1982). *Psychopharmacology of old age.* Oxford, England: Oxford University Press.

6
Functional Psychiatric Disorders in the Elderly

Ira R. Katz, Sharon Curlik, and Paul Nemetz

The functional disorders are the primary problems in general adult psychiatry. They remain important in geriatric psychiatry. The phenomenology, pathogenesis, clinical course, and response to the treatment of these disorders may, however, be altered in the elderly. Furthermore, in work with the elderly, problems commonly arise in the differential diagnosis between organic and functional disorders. When functional disorders occur, they frequently occur in patients with coexisting medical or neurological disease that can obscure diagnosis, complicate treatment, and affect clinical course. Conversely, what appear to be functional disorders may represent, for example, organic, affective, anxiety, or paranoid disorders due to disease of the central nervous system or to less direct effects of somatic disease on the brain. A recurrent theme in both research and clinical work with elderly patients, especially the old-old—those over approximately age 75—and those with chronic physical illness, is the difficulty in distinguishing between the somatic or psychophysiological symptoms of psychiatric disorders and similar symptoms arising from medical illness. In work with the elderly, the discrimination between what is functional and what is, in the wider sense, organic may not be straightforward. The elderly patient with psychiatric symptoms, especially those of late onset, must be thoroughly evaluated for possible medical causes. When psychiatric symptoms or changes in behavior are of sudden onset, medical evaluation is urgent.

I. Depression

A. Epidemiology
  1. Depression is the most common of the functional psychiatric disorders of later life.
  2. Case identification can be difficult in both epidemiological investigation and clinical practice.
      a. Depression is commonly associated with chronic somatic or neurological disease that can obscure the identification of symptoms.
      b. The elderly commonly experience deep, but transient, self-limited depressive states.
      c. The symptomatology of depression may be altered in the elderly.
      d. Losses are common; the distinction between depression and bereavement can be difficult.
  3. There have been several estimates of the prevalence of depression in the community elderly.
      a. Most available estimates are consistent with Blazer and Williams (1980), who reported that 14.7% of the elderly living in the community have a clinically significant degree of dysphoria, 3.7% have major depression (1.8% with primary depression and 1.9% with major depression secondary to other psychiatric disorders), 6.5% have depression associated with significant medical illness, and 4.5% have dysphoria alone.
      b. One set of investigations gives a significantly lower estimate of prevalence (Myers, Weissman, Tischler, et al., 1984). The Epidemiological Catchment Area (ECA) studies utilized a structured interview, the Diagnostic Interview Schedule (DIS), designed to provide *DSM-III* (American Psychiatric Association, 1980) diagnoses. These studies report the six-month prevalence of major depression in the elderly to be 0.1–0.5% for men and 1.0–1.6% for women. There is, however, reason for skepticism in interpreting these findings:
          (1) There was frequent disagreement in the diagnosis of major depression when patients seen by the lay interviewers used for the epidemiological survey were reinterviewed by psychiatrists.
          (2) These studies found a significant decrease with aging in those who reported that they were "ever depressed"; the magnitude of this effect suggests that the methods may not be reliable across all age groups.

(3) The approach used may have discounted depressive symptoms that were similar to effects of drugs or symptoms of somatic disease; thus older patients with depression associated with significant medical illness may have been underestimated.
4. The prevalence is higher in special populations.
   a. In the ambulatory medical care setting, 30-50% of the elderly have significant depressive symptoms. In the acute care hospital, the prevalence is higher.
   b. In long-term care facilities, about 25% of the best-functioning residents have symptoms consistent with a diagnosis of major depression. The prevalence of other dysphoric states (e.g., dysthymic disorder, adjustment reaction with depressed mood) is higher.
5. There may be an effect of aging on the symptomatology of adjustment disorders. Study of the symptoms experienced by medical inpatients suggests that the elderly may be more likely to respond to the stress of hospitalization with depression, while the young may experience more anxiety (Magni & De Leo, 1984).
6. The greater prevalence of depression in women, seen consistently in studies of younger adult populations, may not be seen among the elderly. Prevalence rates become comparable after age 55 to 65; this occurs because rates in women tend to level off, while those in men continue to increase in late life (Weissman & Myers, 1979).
7. Though undertreatment of psychiatric disorders is a problem at all ages, the frequency with which people with depression seek specific treatment declines sharply after age 55 (Weissman & Myers, 1979). Conversely, patients with depressive symptoms have been shown to utilize an excess of medical services for nonspecific complaints.
B. Diagnosis and Symptomatology
   1. The diagnosis of major depression has been validated in the elderly. Other affective disorders and depressive states have been less well investigated.
   2. Major depression with symptoms similar to those seen in younger patients does occur frequently among the elderly. The symptoms of major depression can, however, be altered.
      a. The depressed elderly may be quite reluctant to admit feelings of dysphoria and sadness, such that depression may be "masked" and manifest primarily by somatic concerns (Gurland, 1976). A variety of disturbances, including somatic and autonomic symptoms, pain, hypochondriasis, obsessional

states, and accidents have been proposed as "depressive equivalents." The physician must be alert to the possibility that such symptoms may signal the presence of depression. It is necessary to question patients regarding the presence of the diagnostic symptoms of depression even when complaints of other symptoms are most pressing.
   b. Depression may resemble a state of "depletion" or "disengagement" and may be manifest primarily by apathy, withdrawal, and lack of interest or motivation. Conversely, states of "enervation" related to somatic disease may resemble depression.
   c. The greater problem is under- rather than overdiagnosis of depressive disorders. Valid diagnosis requires that the clinician be familiar with the process of normal aging and be free from "ageist" stereotypes of the inevitability of these symptoms in the elderly.
3. The presence of neurovegetative symptoms of depression (disturbances of sleep, appetite, attention or concentration, psychomotor activity, and energy level) predicts the requirement for antidepressant medications. In the young-old and in those free of significant physical illness, these symptoms remain indicators of major depression. In the more frail elderly and in those with significant physical illness, these symptoms are more ambiguous (Steuer, Bank, Olsen, & Jarvik, 1980; Gurland, Dean, & Cross, 1983).
4. Minimizing the emphasis on somatic and vegetative symptoms may improve the specificity of diagnosis but may do this at the expense of sensitivity. Relying on these symptoms for diagnosis (as with *DSM-III* criteria) may give greater sensitivity at the expense of specificity. Two alternative approaches for dealing with this problem are being developed systematically.
   a. Endicott (1984) has proposed developing and validating diagnostic criteria for major depression that can be applied to patients with specific somatic diseases; in cancer patients, specificity in diagnosis is maintained by placing greater weight on the affective and ideational symptoms relative to the somatic and neurovegetative symptoms of depression.
   b. An essentially opposite approach is implicit in the work of Reifler, Larson, and Hanley (1982), who note that approximately 20% of patients known to have Alzheimer's disease have symptoms consistent with a *DSM-III* diagnosis of major depression. The presence of these symptoms is being used to identify a group of patients to be given therapeutic trials with

antidepressant medication to determine whether they have a treatable component to their disability. This sort of approach may be purposefully overinclusive, sacrificing some degree of specificity for the sake of sensitivity to ensure that patients with disability due in part to depression are not missed.

    c. At present the optimal approach depends on the clinical context. If the goal, for example, is to rule out depression as a treatable source of disability before making a decision about a patient's need for long-term care, it is better to err on the side of overdiagnosis rather than underdiagnosis; in this context, the wider use of therapeutic trials is indicated.

5. Biological markers for depression have not yet been demonstrated to be of practical utility in the diagnosis of depression in the elderly. "False positives" in both the dexamethasone suppression test (Spar, 1982) and the TRH stimulation test (Sunderland, Tariot, Mueller, et al., 1985) can occur in Alzheimer's disease; use of these tests has not been shown to increase the reliability of the diagnosis of depression versus dementia.

6. Major depression with delusions occurs in up to 50% of the elderly hospitalized for depression. There have been suggestions that delusional depression may occur more frequently in older patients, especially in those with initial onset in late life (Myers, 1984).

C. Pathogenesis

1. Several comparisons of elderly depressives with disease of early versus late onset have demonstrated that those with early onset have an excess of depression in first-degree relatives compared to those with late onset. Patients with depression of late onset have an excess of chronic somatic disease. The effects of medical illness may be related to stress reactions, psychological responses to loss of vigor and function, or physiological or metabolic changes in the brain due to either disease or pharmacological treatment.

2. The relevance of the neurochemical and neuroendocrine changes associated with aging (including increases in monoamine oxidase, decreases in catecholamine synthesizing enzymes, alterations in the dynamics of receptor regulation, diminished thyroid function and thyroid responsivity) to the pathogenesis of depression in late life remains speculative (Georgotas, 1983).

3. Psychological Factors

    a. Stressful life events, including losses, contribute strongly to the risk for depression in the aged. There is need for further

research on the distinction between adjustment disorders and more persistent depressive states.
   b. Blau (1983) has reviewed depression in the aged from a psychoanalytic perspective. Reactions to loss, of others or of attributes of the self, are central. The roles of hostile critical feelings being turned against the self, of ego helplessness and conflict within the ego, and of narcissistic vulnerability must be examined within each case. Timing and anticipation of losses can be critical. All would agree that it is necessary but not sufficient to know that a loss occurred. One must learn and understand the particular meaning of the loss to the individual. The psychodynamics of the elderly are an area of intense current inquiry. Developments in this area are of value to all clinicians for understanding the unique situation that each patient represents.
   c. Gallagher and Thompson (1983) have reviewed depression in the aged from the perspective of Beck's cognitive-behavioral theory and have developed effective approaches to time-limited, structured psychotherapeutic treatment based on this model. Depression is viewed as resulting from the negative triad (an interacting set of negative views of oneself, experience, and the future), underlying depressive and depressogenic beliefs or schemata, and such cognitive errors as errors of logic and information processing that maintain the depressed state.
D. Differential Diagnosis
   1. The distinction between irreversible dementia and depression presenting with cognitive impairment is by now a well-recognized problem in differential diagnosis. The term *pseudodementia* has been commonly used; it may, however, be misleading, obscuring the fact that patients with depression may exhibit very real (though treatable) cognitive impairment.
      a. In some patients with depression, functional disability and decreased cognitive performance seem related to a conversion disorder and present as an often-inaccurate caricature of dementia.
      b. In other patients there is a measurable dementia syndrome of depression (Folstein & McHugh, 1978), with cognitive impairment apparent on neuropsychological testing.
      c. The clinical course, the history of previous episodes of depression, and the presence of neurovegetative symptoms may guide diagnosis. Guidelines for clinical diagnosis such as those proposed by Wells (1979) may be useful.

Functional Psychiatric Disorders

      d. Though often proposed as discriminants, recent research has suggested that "I don't know" responses may not, in fact, be more common in depression than in dementia (Young, Manley, & Alexopoulis, 1985).
      e. There is little association between the subjective complaint of memory impairment and the presence or absence of real impairment. Subjective complaints of intellectual deterioration may be more often associated with the diagnosis of depression rather than dementia (Kahn, Zarit, Hilbert, & Niederehe, 1975).
  2. Other problems in differential diagnosis include the distinction between depression and the affective lability of cerebral vascular disease, and the lack of affective expression and decreased motivation of parkinsonism. Frontal lobe syndromes can mimic depression. Primary sleep disorders, with disturbed night-time sleep and excessive daytime sedation, can be confusing. The list of medical and metabolic disturbances (including adverse drug effects) that can cause depression in the elderly is extensive.
  3. It may be difficult to distinguish depression with paranoid delusions and a paranoid disorder with secondary demoralization and depression. A careful history of the onset of the affective, neurovegetative, and delusional symptoms can usually clarify the diagnosis.

E. Treatment and Outcome
  1. The difference between older and younger patients seems to be more in the pharmacokinetics of antidepressant medications than in the pharmacodynamics and in the sensitivity to adverse effects rather than in the nature of the therapeutic response. Monitoring plasma levels of certain antidepressants is more often indicated in the elderly to minimize adverse effects while ensuring adequate treatment.
  2. The drug with well-established plasma level–response correlations that is best tolerated in the elderly is probably nortriptyline. Monoamine oxidase (MAO) inhibitors can be both safe and effective in the elderly, provided that precautions regarding diet and drug interactions are followed. The efficacy of treatment could be improved through routine laboratory monitoring of the treatment-related inhibition of platelet MAO. Electroconvulsive therapy is still the most effective treatment for severe depression. Delusional depression is likely to require either electroconvulsive therapy or a combination of neuroleptic and antidepressant medication, although the former treatment is believed to be more efficacious.

3. The value of psychotherapy for depression in the aged has been established. Even in the elderly, if patients do not respond to any form of adequate treatment within 6 to 8 weeks, alternative approaches must be considered.
4. Affective disorders are as a rule recurrent. Depression occurring in late life is a disorder requiring long-term follow-up and treatment. Post (1972) followed 92 patients hospitalized and treated for depression and observed that 26% of the survivors made a sustained recovery, 37% had a recurrence with subsequent recovery, 25% had recurrent attacks in the setting of chronic, mild depression, and 12% were continuously ill throughout the period of follow-up. More recently Murphy (1983) observed that 42% of the survivors from a mixed group of depressed inpatients and outpatients were well when followed up at 1 year, 23% had improved but then relapsed, and 35% were continuously ill. Factors associated with poor prognosis included the presence of delusions during the initial episode, poor health, and psychosocial stress occurring during the follow-up period. Follow-up of elderly patients admitted to the hospital for treatment of depression has not demonstrated an excess in the incidence of dementia (Roth, 1955).
5. There are clear associations between depression and functional disability. Though depression can represent an affective barrier to rehabilitation, there is, at present, little evidence allowing discrimination between depression as a cause, and depression as a result, of disability. Depressed patients have been shown to have poorer social supports than age-matched controls. Community adjustment and the perceived quality of social relations improve with the resolution of depressive symptoms.
6. Evaluating the response to treatment can be difficult, especially in patients with depression coexisting with medical or neurological disease. These problems are corollaries of the difficulties in diagnosis.
    a. When patients do not respond to treatment, or when they respond with only partial resolution of depressive symptoms and functional disability, it is important to evaluate the adequacy of current treatment, to consider the probable safety and efficacy of additive or alternative approaches, and to reevaluate the diagnosis.
        (1) For patients with a definite diagnosis of major depression, the treating physician should use all available approaches to ensure and maintain relief from symptoms.

(2) When treatment is initiated in patients with a questionable diagnosis to test the possibility that depression was contributing to disability, careful clinical judgment is required to decide when a failure to respond is an indication for an alternative approach to treatment and when it is an indication that depression was not a significant cause of impairment. Though we cannot expect a therapeutic trial of antidepressant medication to give a definitive answer in every instance, one of the goals of such a trial is to be able to assure nonresponding patients and their caretakers that treatable sources of impairment have been excluded and that adaptation to persistent disability is necessary.
   b. Sorensen, Kragh-Sorenson, Larson, & Hvidberg (1978) reported that 80-90% of patients with major depression responded to nortriptyline treatment when dosage was adjusted to achieve plasma drug levels of 60-150 ng/ml. With other available agents, adequate treatment is either not as well tolerated or not as well defined. In the absence of medical contraindications, nortriptyline may presently be the agent of first choice for the treatment of depression in the aged and the most appropriate medication for the conduct of therapeutic trials.
F. Mortality
   1. Depression in the elderly is associated with increased mortality. This finding holds in both patient populations and in subjects found to have depressive symptoms in community surveys (Enzell, 1984). Depression is associated with a high rate of suicide, but the increased mortality is observed even when suicide is excluded. Though depression may be an early manifestation of occult neoplasm, the increased mortality holds even when death from cancer is excluded. Similar findings were reported both in recent studies and in studies conducted in the 1930s; the cause of excess deaths cannot be attributed to adverse effects of antidepressant medication.
   2. The causes for the higher death rate include cardiovascular and cerebrovascular disease. Given that depression with late onset is associated with an excess of chronic somatic disease, it is possible that the increased mortality is not directly related to the depressive state but is rather a reflection of the greater frailty of the depressed population. However, the higher death rate applies for both early and late onset depression. Depressed patients with cardiovascular disease have increased mortality. However,

depressed patients have higher rates of myocardial infarction. Most significantly, there is data suggesting that mortality in depression is decreased in patients who receive adequate treatment (Avery & Winokur, 1976). Thus there is evidence that recognition and treatment of depression in the elderly can prolong life as well as improve its quality. Possible mechanisms for the excess mortality include decreased self-care, neuroendocrine dysregulation, malnutrition, and impaired immune function.

G. Suicide
  1. Suicide rates increase with increasing age in both men and women. Though there are, no doubt, significant cohort effects, this trend has repeatedly been observed cross-nationally and cross-culturally.
  2. Elderly white males are the demographic group with the highest incidence of suicide. Rates for white males 60 and older in this country are 40–75 per year per 100,000, compared to 9–13 per year per 100,000 for the entire older population. Rates for men are on the order of five times the rates in women.
  3. Suicide attempts are, in general, serious in the elderly. The ratio of suicide attempts to successful suicides has been estimated as 4-to-1 in the elderly, compared to 20-to-1 in those under age 40.
  4. Risk factors for suicide include physical illness, previous attempts or gestures, bereavement, and isolation and loneliness, as well as psychiatric disorders. It has been estimated that 50–70% of late-life suicides have had significant depression.

II. Mania and Bipolar Disorder

A. Epidemiology
  1. The prevalence of mania is quite low among the elderly in the community. It has been estimated that it is the basis for 5–10% of clinical referrals for treatment of affective disorder. Roth (1955) found that 13% of patients admitted for inpatient treatment of affective disorder had predominantly manic symptomatology.
  2. Post and colleagues (Cutler & Post, 1982) have suggested that the natural history of bipolar disorder involves increases in the frequency and duration of recurrences, a decrease in the period between episodes, and an increase in the prevalence of rapid cycling as a function of both aging and the duration of illness.
  3. Though the initial occurrence of mania in the seventh or eighth decades is rare, it has been reported both in affective disorders of late onset and, in disorders of early onset, as much as 50 years after the initial occurrence of depression.

4. The onset of mania in late life, however, should raise the possibility that it is a symptomatic state rather than a primary affective disorder; it should trigger investigations for possible organic causes from structural neurological disease, from adverse effects of medications, or from medical or metabolic disease.
B. Diagnosis and Symptomatology
   1. Mania is probably underdiagnosed in the elderly, largely because manic episodes are frequently atypical in late life (Shulman & Post, 1980).
      a. Mania is less often characterized by pure and infectious states of elation. The affect is more often aggressive, angry, and irritable. Mixed states with considerable dysphoria are common.
      b. Hyperactivity may be muted. Mania may resemble agitated depression or states of catatonia.
      c. Hostile and suspicious thought content is more common than expansive delusions of wealth and power.
      d. Confusion is common; mania as well as depression can mimic dementia.
      e. Vigilance regarding atypical presentations of mania and bipolar disease may be most important in evaluating depressed patients who do not respond to, or who appear to worsen with, antidepressant treatment.
C. Recognition of manic states in the elderly, as in the young, suggests the need for lithium treatment. Even in late life, lithium remains the cornerstone for the treatment and prophylaxis of mania. It is, of course, necessary to carefully monitor the older patient for confusion, ataxia, and decreased renal function. The older patient may be at increased risk for both cognitive impairment and nephrotoxicity. Neuroleptics remain useful for the management of acute episodes. The safety and efficacy of carbamazepine for treatment of bipolar illness in the elderly remains to be established. Its use should, however, be considered in patients who are intolerant or unresponsive to lithium.

III. Functional Psychoses

A. Psychoses of Late Onset
   1. The functional psychoses of late onset are almost invariably of a paranoid nature.
   2. There is concern that the psychoses of late onset were not dealt with adequately in *DSM-III* (Volavka, 1985).
      a. *DSM-III* provides for the diagnosis of paranoid disorders characterized by jealous or persecutory delusions with no promi-

nent hallucinations and no incoherence, loose associations, or bizarre delusions as would be present in schizophrenia.
   b. Psychoses with prominent hallucinations and schizophrenia-like symptoms do occur with onset in late life (Bridge & Wyatt, 1980a,b). Some of these are indistinguishable in terms of symptoms from paranoid schizophrenia. Nevertheless, *DSM-III* (1980) specifically excludes the diagnosis of schizophrenia when psychotic symptoms begin after age 45. The more current revised *DSM-III-R* (1987) does recognize the possibility that schizophrenia may begin in late life.
   c. The functional psychoses of late onset may not, however, be adequately described with these diagnoses. At present, it appears useful to rely upon Roth's concept of "late paraphrenia" in discussing these disorders.
3. Late paraphrenia: Work by Roth (1955) provided validation for the concept of late paraphrenia by demonstrating that it could be distinguished in terms of both symptoms and prognosis from patients with depression and dementia. Post's (1966) experience with a series of 93 consecutive inpatients with late paraphrenia suggested three types of paraphrenic disorders.
   a. Simple paranoid psychosis: Delusional ideas are limited in content to one or two themes, mainly concerning the patient's relationship with neighbors and, less commonly, relatives. There are frequently auditory or olfactory hallucinations with related content. The psychotic content is usually persecutory or jealous, but almost always commonplace. This represented 24% of the patients in Post's series. It is probably the most common of these disorders, but, because it is the one with the least pervasive and least disruptive symptoms, it is the least likely to come to psychiatric attention.
   b. Schizophrenia-like illness: Content is paranoid, often banal, but quite pervasive and disruptive. Patients become increasingly distressed by hallucinatory experiences and paranoid delusions, which are only loosely connected. They can become panicky or aggressive in response to threatening voices or perceived persecutors. Schneiderian symptoms are absent. This state was seen in 40% of patients.
   c. Paranoid schizophrenia: The symptoms include Schneiderian first-rank symptoms, commonly third-person-singular auditory hallucinations, but also delusions of influence, passivity, thought broadcasting, and thought insertion. This is the most severe and most disabling form of late paraphrenia. It was seen in 36% of patients.

4. Epidemiology
   a. Christenson and Blazer (1984) found the prevalence of generalized persecutory ideation in a random community sample to be 4%. Half of these were in subjects with cognitive impairment, reducing the prevalence of functional paranoid psychoses to approximately 2%.
   b. Functional psychoses of late onset have been reported to represent 3-10% of first psychiatric admission in the elderly. Clinical studies consistently find an excess of late onset psychoses in women.
   c. *DSM-III* paranoid disorders appear to be far less common.
5. Differential Diagnosis
   a. Paranoid disorders of late life must be distinguished from chronic schizophrenia and mania.
   b. The distinction between paraphrenia and delusional depression can usually be made on the basis of history and the intensity of the affective symptoms.
   c. Symptoms similar to those of paraphrenia can result from metabolic disorders and drug toxicity.
   d. Paranoid psychosis can occur as a common complication of dementing illness. When present, it can represent a treatable component to the patient's distress and the caretaker's burden. Conversely, the late-onset psychoses can occur with deterioration in functional status and self-care as well as poor performance on cognitive testing; these disorders can mimic dementia.
   e. Late paraphrenics should be distinguished from senile recluses, nonpsychotic individuals characterized by eccentric behavior, secretiveness, and isolation; these patients frequently come into medical contact as a result of deterioration due to self-neglect.
6. Pathogenesis
   a. Late paraphrenia appears to be loosely related to schizophrenia on genetic grounds. The risk for developing schizophrenia in siblings and children of late paraphrenics is intermediate between that of early-onset schizophrenics and the general population (approximately 3.4% vs. 5.8% and 0.8%, respectively).
   b. Only 10-30% of patients are characterized by their relatives or friends as having been "normal" before the onset of their illness. The illness appears to develop slowly out of a deviant or eccentric personality; premorbid personality has been characterized as quarrelsome-aggressive-hostile, egocentric-

obstinant-domineering, suspicious-jealous-persecuted, or shy-sensitive-withdrawn. Work records are often good, but there is commonly a failure of closer interpersonal relationships, shown especially by low marriage rates and late marriage (Kay, Cooper, Garside, & Roth, 1976).
   c. Sensory impairment, especially social deafness, is a risk factor. Though visual defects are probably more common in paraphrenia than in depression, the etiological significance of visual impairment is not as well established. There does not appear to be a significant relationship with chronic somatic disease.
   d. Recent work has utilized CT scanning to demonstrate "occult" organic lesions in a group of patients with symptoms of late-onset paraphrenia (Miller, Benson, Cummings, & Neshkes, 1986). Further research utilizing current techniques for brain imaging is necessary to test the hypothesis that late paraphrenia may frequently be an organic delusional syndrome.
7. Treatment and Outcome
   a. Though patients with dementia rather commonly experience paranoid symptoms, late paraphrenia is not, in general, a prodrome of dementia (Roth, 1955).
   b. Patients with simple paranoid states and those with schizophrenia-like illness, but not those with first-rank symptoms, may lose their active symptoms, at least temporarily, when transferred from relative isolation to a more structured and supportive environment.
   c. All patients with persecutory symptoms should be evaluated for sensory impairment; hearing and visual deficits should be corrected.
   d. The paraphrenias, in general, respond to acute treatment with antipsychotic medication with the elimination, or at least a reduction, in symptoms; most patients can be discharged from the hospital.
   e. Most patients require maintenance treatment to prevent recurrence and disability. The most powerful predictor of successful outcome is compliance with maintenance pharmacotherapy. Use of depot neuroleptics makes adequate treatment more accessible to these patients.
   f. There have been suggestions that *DSM-III* paranoid disorder may be less responsive to antipsychotic medication than the paraphrenias in general. Given the lack of extensive data on this rather rare condition, it is at present reasonable to sug-

Functional Psychiatric Disorders 127

gest that all psychotic patients should be given the benefit of a trial of antipsychotic medication.

B. Chronic Schizophrenia
1. The prevalence of chronic schizophrenia has been estimated as 0.3–1.0% of the elderly in the community. In this country, approximately 35% of nursing home residents are chronic schizophrenic patients. Though schizophrenics of all ages are in nursing homes, 90% of them are over age 65.
2. Schizophrenic patients who survive into late life are a heterogeneous group varying in terms of the chronicity of symptoms, the length of institutionalization, and treatment history. Their capacities and needs reflect both the natural history of their disease, the impact of treatment and institutionalization, and the impact of available social supports. The first cohorts of schizophrenics whose illness developed after effective treatment became available are only now coming of age. The nature of this group continues to evolve as a function of developments in psychopharmacology, community psychiatry, and programs for deinstitutionalization over the past 30 years.
3. Information on elderly chronic schizophrenics is available primarily from studies on the long-term outcome of schizophrenia.
    a. The available data suggest a positive effect of aging on at least a subgroup of schizophrenic patients (Lawton, 1972; Bleuler, 1974; Ciompi, 1980).
    b. In viewing these findings, however, it is important to note that patients with the most severe illnesses are less likely to have survived into old age.
    c. By age 60, symptoms of schizophrenia are often more subdued and less disruptive. Positive symptoms are often less intense; hallucinations and delusions are less compelling or more easily concealed. The symptoms that allow subtyping of schizophrenia are less prominent in elderly chronic patients, and distinctions between subtypes appear to be lost.
    d. The effect of aging on schizophrenia is not simply an amelioration of positive symptoms. Negative, deficit symptoms may improve in late life. The older schizophrenic may improve with respect to affect, motivation, and social responsivity.
4. There is little data to guide the clinician in the treatment of the aged chronic schizophrenic. Clearly the need for maintenance treatment should be reassessed in the elderly patient when aging or age-related disease (tardive dyskinesia, parkinsonism, abnormalities of gait, cardiovascular disease, cognitive dysfunction, etc.) alters the risk/benefit ratio for use of antipsychotic medica-

tions. Similarly, the age-related changes in symptomatology should encourage the intensification of psychosocial approaches to treatment and rehabilitation.

IV. Anxiety Disorders

A. The anxiety disorders of late life have not been intensively investigated. There has been little clinical research based on operationally defined diagnoses as described in *DSM-III*. However, the literature on neuroses in the elderly is clearly relevant. A recurrent problem in both research and clinical practice is the coexistence of anxiety with depression and the difficulty, especially in the elderly, in distinguishing between anxiety and depressive disorders (Roth & Mountjoy, 1980).
B. Epidemiology
  1. Up to 10% or 15% of the elderly have neurotic or personality disorders.
  2. Bergmann (1971) compared older patients with "neurotic" symptoms of early versus late onset. Patients with late-onset disorders had experienced more social isolation and physical illness, particularly cardiovascular disease. The patients with late onset were more likely to have predominantly depressive symptoms, while those with early onset were more likely to have predominantly anxiety.
  3. Himmelfarb and Murrell (1984) demonstrated that 17% of males and 22% of females had anxiety of a degree that warranted treatment; the prevalence is higher in the old-old. Though anxiolytic agents are, no doubt, frequently overprescribed and overused, distressing and disabling anxiety disorders may frequently go untreated because of both patient and physician bias against treatment.
  4. Panic disorder with onset in late life appears to be rather uncommon; when panic attacks occur for the first time in late life it is important to look for both organic causes and symptoms of underlying depression.
  5. Phobic symptoms are difficult to evaluate; it is unclear how frequently the rather mundane fears that lead to restriction of activities in the elderly (e.g., not going out after dark or when there is ice on the ground) can be viewed as phobias.
  6. Obsessive-compulsive disorder is uncommon in the aged. When obsessions or compulsions occur with onset in late life, they are likely to be symptoms of other disorders (e.g., they may be depressive equivalents).

7. Generalized anxiety disorder must be distinguished from situational, often self-limited adjustment disorders with anxious mood.
C. Diagnosis and symptomatology: The symptoms of anxiety states in the elderly are, in general, similar to those of generalized anxiety in the young. Somatic and psychophysiological symptoms (headache, palpitations, abdominal symptoms, and insomnia) are common; they may be difficult to distinguish from symptoms of physical illness. Hypochondriacal symptoms are common, but derealization and depersonalization are rare.
D. Differential diagnosis: Anxiety can be a primary disorder or a symptom of almost any psychiatric disorder, organic or functional. The evaluation of the anxious patient must include the evaluation of cognitive status to rule out delirium and dementia. Medical and metabolic causes of anxiety can be diverse; they include drug effects, withdrawal from sedative-hypnotic medications, caffeinism, hyperthyroidism, hypoglycemia, and cardiac and pulmonary disorders.
E. Outcome
   1. Anxiety disorders in late life are frequently chronic, or characterized by recurrent symptoms.
   2. Long-term studies of outcome show morbidity both in terms of symptoms and social adaptation. Little is known of the impact of treatment on long-term course.
   3. States of anxiety can be associated with impairment in cognitive performance.
   4. There have been few studies in the aged of the interrelationships between anxiety and functional status or of the impact of anxiety on health and mortality. Without such data it is difficult to evaluate the risks versus the benefits of the use of anxiolytic medications.
   5. The elderly are at increased risk for adverse effects of benzodiazepines prescribed for treatment of anxiety. When these medications are prescribed, they should be used in time-limited courses of treatment, with regular monitoring of therapeutic benefit as well as side effects. Long-acting benzodiazepines (e.g., diazepam, chlordiazepoxide) are likely to accumulate with time in the older patient, with increased risk for cognitive impairment, daytime sedation, dizziness, and ataxia. Doses of short-acting benzodiazepines (e.g., oxazepam, lorazepam, alprazolam) can be more easily titrated; these agents are, in general, preferable for treatment of the older patient.

V. Alcoholism

Alcoholism and the misuse of sedative-hypnotic medication, frequently iatrogenic, constitute the most significant types of substance abuse in the elderly. Abuse of analgesics and anti-inflammatory agents, however, is also common and can lead to confusion, gastrointestinal disease, and renal disease.

A. Epidemiology
   1. Estimates of the prevalence of alcoholism in the community elderly are on the order of 2-10% (Schuckit, 1982).
   2. The prevalence among patients seeking medical care is higher, approximately 10-15%.
   3. A study of elderly medical and surgical admissions to a VA hospital demonstrated that 20% of patients had a lifetime diagnosis of alcoholism. Almost half had been actively drinking prior to hospitalization.
   4. Alcoholism is associated with a high mortality; death from cirrhosis peaks at ages 55-64. Thus older alcoholics with early onset of drinking may be a select group of survivors. Older patients who have "matured out" of alcoholism may be commonly seen if history-taking is adequate. The fate of these patients remains to be established.
   5. Among men, as many as 25% report heavy drinking in their early sixties; the number decreases to 6-7% in the seventies. Patients with alcoholism of late onset represent about 10% of alcoholics admitted for treatment.

B. Diagnosis and Symptomatology
   1. Classical signs of alcohol dependence, intoxication, or withdrawal are often not evident in the elderly. Instead, there may be less specific presentations, such as confusion, poor hygiene, falls, incontinence, myopathy, poor nutrition, and accidental hypothermia.
   2. These symptoms may be misdiagnosed as due to dementia or functional disability secondary to somatic disease. When major problems include erratic or paranoid behavior, family difficulties or estrangement, primary alcoholism may be confused with other psychiatric disorders.
   3. In the elderly, as in the young, 5-15% of alcoholism is secondary to other preexisting psychiatric disorders, primarily depression. In the elderly, alcoholism of late onset is more likely to be secondary to depression.
   4. The *DSM-III* diagnosis of alcoholism requires evidence of pathological (excessive) use and impairment in social or vocational

functioning. The slower metabolism and increased tissue sensitivity to the pathological effects of alcohol make it difficult to define "excessive" use in the elderly in quantitative terms. Decreased vocational demands and the tendency for the older patient to be protected by social and environmental supports may make it difficult to identify alcohol-related functional impairment (Schuckit, 1978).
   5. Elderly alcoholics are more likely to drink on a daily basis than the young. Their daily intake, however, is lower, averaging four drinks per day.
C. Outcome and Treatment
   1. Even when alcoholics of late onset have a benign social course, they may have a malignant medical outcome. Elderly alcoholics exhibit increased mortality with risk for gastrointestinal, cardiac, and pulmonary disease; falls; and dementia.
   2. There is a high risk for both secondary depression and dementia.
   3. Alcoholism in late life is characterized by exacerbations and remissions.
   4. Prognosis is improved for alcoholics who become abstinent, and active approaches to treatment are important.
   5. There has been little research on the treatment of the elderly alcoholic. As with the younger patient, treatment should consist of:
      a. Evaluation of the need for detoxification.
      b. Rehabilitation in the inpatient setting, an intensive outpatient program, or in the context of psychotherapy.
      c. Referral to Alcoholics Anonymous or similar programs.
      d. Antabuse (disulfiram) can be a valuable adjunct to psychosocial treatment. Its safety and efficacy should be further examined, specifically in the elderly.

VI. Sleep and Sleep Disorders

A. Though significant changes in the sleep/wake cycle are consistently found in studies of normal aging, the elderly vary extensively in both sleep parameters and in their subjective response to these changes (Weitzman, 1983). Sleep changes in the normal aged include:
   1. Nighttime sleep is, in general, shortened, with multiple brief awakenings.
   2. There is a shift of one to two hours earlier (phase advance) in the time of going to sleep.

3. Changes observed in sleep EEG include:
   a. A decrease in time spent in stage 4 (high amplitude, slow wave) sleep.
   b. A decrease in total REM sleep time, but no change in the fraction of total sleep time spent in REM.
   c. A shortening of the first REM cycle, probably related to the decrease in stage 4 sleep occurring before the first REM period (in this respect, the sleep changes in normal aging can resemble those in depression).

B. Sleep Disturbances in the Elderly
   1. Experience in sleep laboratories has indicated that objective findings of specific sleep disorders are more common, and significant psychopathology is less common in older patients presenting for evaluation.
   2. Young patients appear to complain more often about difficulty in initiating sleep, while older patients seem to complain more frequently about difficulty in maintaining sleep, including early awakenings.
   3. Kripke, Simons, and Garfinkle (1979) reviewed epidemiological data from an American Cancer Society study demonstrating that sleep disturbances are associated with significant increases in mortality.
      a. Subjects who reported that they slept fewer than 7 or more than 7.9 hours each night were observed to exhibit increased mortality over a six-year follow-up period.
      b. Subjects who stated they used sleeping medication often were 50% more likely to die during follow-up than those who never used sleeping medication.
      c. Elderly subjects were highly overrepresented in those with extremely long and extremely short sleep duration.
      d. In the elderly, mortality was doubled for those who slept fewer than 4 or more than 10 hours per night (relative to those who slept 7.5 hours).
   4. The most common primary sleep disorders in the aged are the sleep apnea syndromes and periodic movements in sleep (nocturnal myoclonus) (Coleman et al., 1981; Roehrs, Zorick, Sicklesteel, Witting, & Roth, 1983). In a community sample assessed with in-home monitoring, 62% of the sample showed evidence for apneas and/or leg myoclonus during sleep (18% had apneas; 34%, leg jerks; and 10%, both) in spite of the fact that 80% of the sample reported satisfactory sleep (Ancoli-Israel, Kripke, Mason, & Kaplan, 1985). The significance of these pathological findings in community subjects remains to be established.

a. Sleep apnea
   (1) Occurs in 25-40% of elderly patients evaluated in sleep centers.
   (2) Is manifest as both a disorder of initiating and maintaining sleep and as a disorder of excessive daytime somnolence.
   (3) Can occur in both central and obstructive forms; the disorder in the elderly is, in general, of mixed type. Loud snoring is a useful, though not a universal, marker for the disorder.
   (4) Increases in prevalence with age and obesity. It is more common in men.
   (5) Is a disorder with a high mortality. It may be a common cause of death occurring during sleep. It is likely the primary cause of the mortality associated with sleep disturbances in the elderly as noted by Kripke.
   (6) Is exacerbated (both the frequency and severity of apneas is increased) by sedative-hypnotic medications. Use of such medications by elderly patients with sleep apnea can be lethal.
   (7) May present with symptoms of insomnia and decreased energy, motivation, and activities; it may be confused with a retarded depression.
   (8) Changes in sleep EEG and disordered breathing in sleep appear to be common in patients with Alzheimer's disease and related to the degree of cognitive impairment; their clinical significance is not yet established (Prinz et al., 1982; Reynolds et al., 1985).
b. Periodic movement during sleep (nocturnal myoclonus)
   (1) Occurs in 20-30% of elderly patients evaluated in sleep centers.
   (2) Is most frequently manifested as a disorder of initiating and maintaining sleep, and less commonly occurs as a disorder of excessive daytime somnolence. The movements are in general accompanied by brief arousals; the patient may or may not be aware of them.

C. Treatment
   1. In general, sedative-hypnotic medication should be used only for limited periods of time, as for the short-term management of situational insomnia.
   2. Sedative-hypnotic medications are commonly prescribed for the elderly, especially those in the acute hospital or long-term care facility, without diagnosis of the nature of the patient's sleep

disturbance. They are frequently prescribed for a period of time that far exceeds their established efficacy. Problems resulting include exacerbation of sleep disturbances as a result of drug tolerance and worsening of sleep apnea in addition to the side effects of the specific agent used.
3. Treatment for persistent sleep disturbances must be based on the specific diagnosis. Referral to the sleep laboratory may frequently be necessary. A practical method for in-home screening for sleep apnea syndromes would greatly facilitate diagnosis.
   a. Sleep apnea: Nasal continuous positive airway pressure (CPAP) has probably replaced tracheostomy as the treatment of choice for moderate to severe obstructive apneas. Weight loss can be effective. ENT examination for specific anatomic causes for obstruction should be routine. The role of psychopharmacological treatment (e.g., acetazolamide, protriptyline) has not been well established.
   b. Nocturnal myoclonus: Clonazepam is the best established treatment for nocturnal myoclonus. The risks of its use in the elderly are similar to those of other long-acting benzodiazepines. It is not clear whether it acts by decreasing the arousal associated with periodic movements or whether it decreases the movements themselves. The relative efficacy of other benzodiazepines (including shorter-acting benzodiazepines) requires further investigation.

REFERENCES

American Psychiatric Association. (1980). *Diagnostic and statistical manual of mental disorders* (3rd ed.). Washington, DC: American Psychiatric Press.

American Psychiatric Association. (1987). *Diagnostic and statistical manual of mental disorders* (3d ed., revised). Washington, DC: American Psychiatric Press.

Ancoli-Israel, S., Kripke, D. F., Mason, W., & Kaplan, O. J. (1985). Sleep apnea and periodic movements in an aging sample. *J Gerontology, 40,* 419–425.

Avery, D., & Winokur, G. (1976). Mortality in depressed patients treated with electroconvulsive therapy and antidepressants. *Arch Gen Psychiatry, 33,* 1029–1037.

Bergmann, K. (1971). The neuroses of old age. In D. W. K. Kay & A. Walk (Eds.), Recent developments in psychogeriatrics. *Br J Psychiatry* (Special Publication No. 6), 35–90.

Blau, D. (1983). Depression in the elderly: A psychoanalytical perspective. In L. D. Breslau & M. R. Haug (Eds.), *Depression and aging* (pp. 75–93). New York: Springer.

Blazer, D., & Williams, C. D. (1980). Epidemiology of dysphoria and depression in an elderly population. *Amer J Psychiatry, 139,* 439-444.

Bleuler, M. (1974). The long-term course of the schizophrenic psychoses. *Psychol Med, 4,* 244-254.

Bridge, T. P., & Wyatt, R. J. (1980a). Paraphrenia: Paranoid states of late life. I. European Research. *J Am Ger Soc, 28,* 193-200.

Bridge, T. P., & Wyatt, R. J. (1980b). Paraphrenia: Paranoid states of late life. II. American Research. *J Am Ger Soc, 28,* 201-205.

Christenson, R., & Blazer, D. (1984). Epidemiology of persecutory ideation in an elderly population in the community. *Amer J Psychiatry, 141,* 1088-1091.

Ciompi, L. (1980). Catamnesic long-term study on the course of life and aging of schizophrenics. *Schiz Bull, 6,* 606-618.

Coleman, R. M., Miles, L. E., Guilleminault, C. C., Zarcone, V. P., Vanden Hood, J., & Dement, W. C. (1981). Sleep-wake disorders in the elderly: A polysomnographic analysis. *J Am Ger Soc, 7,* 289-296.

Cutler, N. R., & Post, R. M. (1982). Life course of illness in untreated manic depressive patients. *Comp Psychiatry, 23,* 101-115.

Endicott, J. (1984). Measurement of depression in patients with cancer. *Cancer, 53,* 2243-2248.

Enzell, K. (1984). Mortality among persons with depressive symptoms and among responders and non-responders in a health check-up. *Acta Psychiatr Scand, 69,* 89-102.

Folstein, M. F., & McHugh, P. R. (1978). Dementia syndrome of depression. In R. Katzman, R. Terry, & K. L. Bick (Eds.), *Alzheimer's disease: Senile dementia and related disorders* (pp. 87-93). New York: Raven.

Gallagher, D., & Thompson, L. W. (1983). Cognitive therapy for depression in the elderly: A promising model for treatment and research. In L. D. Breslau & M. R. Haug (Eds.), *Depression and aging* (pp. 168-192). New York: Springer.

Georgotas, A. (1983). Affective disorders in the elderly: Diagnostic and research considerations. *Age and Aging, 12,* 1-10.

Gurland, B. J. (1976). The comparative frequency of depression in various adult age groups. *J Gerontol, 31,* 283-292.

Gurland, B. J., Dean, L. L., & Cross, P. S. (1983). The effects of depression on individual social functioning in the elderly. In L. D. Breslau & M. R. Haug (Eds.), *Depression and aging* (pp. 256-265). New York: Springer.

Himmelfarb, S., & Murrell, S. A. (1984). The prevalence and correlates of anxiety symptoms in older adults. *J Psychology, 116,* 159-167.

Kahn, R. L., Zarit, S. H., Hilbert, N. M., & Niederehe, G. (1975). Memory complaint and impairment in the aged. *Arch Gen Psychiatry, 32,* 1569-1573.

Kay, D. W. K., Cooper, H. F., Garside, R. F., & Roth, M. (1976). The differentiation of paranoid from affective psychoses by patients' premorbid characteristics. *Br J Psychiatry, 129,* 207-215.

Kripke, D., Simons, R., & Garfinkel, L. (1979). Short and long sleep and sleeping pills. *Arch Gen Psychiatry, 36,* 103-116.

Lawton, M. P. (1972). Schizophrenia forty-five years later. *J Genet Psychol., 121,* 133-143.

Magni, D., & De Leo, D. (1984). Anxiety and depression in geriatric and adult medical inpatients: A comparison. *Psychol Rep, 55,* 607-612.

Miller, B. L., Benson, F., Cummings, J., & Neshkes, R. (1986). Late-life paraphrenia: An organic delusional syndrome. *J Clin Psychiatry, 47,* 204-207.

Murphy, E. (1983). The prognosis of depression in old age. *Br J Psychiatry, 142,* 111-119.

Myers, B. F., Kalayum, B., & Mei-Tal, V. (1984). Late-onset delusional depression: A distinct clinical entity? *J Clin Psychiatry, 45,* 347-349.

Myers, J. K., Weissman, M. M., Tischler, G. L., Holzer, C. E., Leat, P. J., Orvaschel, H., Anthony, J. C., Boyd, J. H., Burke, J. D., Kramer, M., & Stoltzman, R. (1984). Six-month prevalence of psychiatric disorders in the community. *Arch Gen Psychiatry, 41,* 959-967.

Post, F. (1966). *Persistent persecutory states of the elderly.* Oxford, England: Pergamon.

Post, F. (1972). The management and nature of depressive illness in late life: A follow-through study. *Br J Psychiatry, 212,* 393-404.

Prinz, P. H., Peskind, E. R., Vitaliano, P. P., Raskind, M. A., Eisdorfer, C., Zemcuznikow, N., & Gerber, C. J. (1982). Changes in the sleep and waking EEGs of nondemented and demented elderly subjects. *J Am Ger Soc, 30,* 86-93.

Reynolds, C. F., Kupfer, D. J., Taska, L. S., Hoch, C. C., Sewitch, D. E., Restito, K., Spiker, D. G., Zimmer, B., Marin, R. S., Nelson, J., Martin, D., & Morycz, R. (1985). Sleep apnea in Alzheimer's dementia: Correlation with mental deterioration. *J Clin Psychiatry, 46,* 257-261.

Reifler, B. V., Larson, E., & Hanley, R. (1982). Coexistence of cognitive impairment and depression in geriatric outpatients. *Amer J Psychiatry, 139,* 623-626.

Roehrs, T., Zorick, F., Sicklesteel, J., Witting, R., & Roth, T. (1983). Age-related sleep-wake disorders at a sleep disorder center. *J Am Ger Soc, 31,* 364-370.

Roth, M. (1955). The natural history of mental disorders in old age. *J Ment Sci, 101,* 281-301.

Roth, M., & Mountjoy, C. (1981). States of anxiety in late life; Prevalence of anxiety and related disorders in the elderly. In G. D. Burrows & S. B. Davies (Eds.), *Handbook of studies on anxiety.* New York: Elsevier.

Schuckit, M. A. (1978). The elderly as a unique population: Alcoholism. *Alcoholism: Clin Exp Res, 2,* 31-38.

Schuckit, M. A. (1982). A clinical review of alcohol, alcoholism and the elderly patient. *J Clin Psychiatry, 43,* 396-399.

Shulman, K., & Post, F. (1980). Bipolar affective disorder in old age. *Br J Psychiatry, 136,* 26-32.

Sorensen, B., Kragh-Sorensen, P., Larsen, N. E., & Hvidberg, E. F. (1978). The practical significance of nortriptyline plasma level control. *Psychopharmacology, 59*(1), 35-9, 15.

Spar, J. E. (1982). Does the dexamethasone suppression test distinguish dementia from depression? *Amer J Psychiatry, 139,* 238-240.

Steuer, J., Bank, L., Olsen, E. J., & Jarvik, L. F. (1980). Depression, physical

health, and somatic complaints in the elderly: A study of the Zung Self-Rating Depression Scale. *J Gerontol, 35,* 683-688.
Sunderland, T., Tariot, P. N., Mueller, E. A., Newhouse, P. A., Murphy, D. L., & Cohen, R. M. (1985). TRH stimulation of test in dementia of the Alzheimer type and elderly controls. *Psychiatric Res, 16,* 269-275.
Volavka, J. (1985). Late-onset schizophrenia: A review. *Comp Psychiatry, 26,* 148-156.
Weissman, M. M., & Myers, J. K. (1979). Depression in the elderly: Research directions in psychopathology, epidemiology, and treatment. *J Geriatric Psychiatry, 12,* 187-201.
Weitzman, E. D. (1983). Sleep and aging. In R. Katzman & R. Terry (Eds.), *The neurology of aging* (pp. 167-188). Philadelphia: Davis.
Wells, C. E. (1979). Pseudodementia. *Amer J Psychiatry, 136,* 895-900.
Young, R. C., Manley, M. W., & Alexopoulis, G. S. (1985). "I don't know" responses in elderly depressives and in dementia. *J Amer Ger Soc, 33,* 253-257.

ADDITIONAL READINGS

Birren, J. E., & Sloane, R. B. (1980). *Handbook of mental health and aging.* Englewood Cliffs, NJ: Prentice-Hall.
Blazer, D. G. (1982). *Depression in late life.* St. Louis, MO: Mosby.
Breslau, L. D. & Haug, M. R. (1983). *Depression and aging.* New York: Springer.
Busse, E. W., & Blazer, D. G. (1980). *Handbook of geriatric psychiatry.* New York: Van Nostrand Reinhold.
Jarvik, L. F., & Small, G. W. (1982). *Psychiatric clinics of North America: Vol. 5.* Philadelphia: W. B. Saunders.
Kaplan, O. J. (1979). *Psychopathology of aging.* New York: Academic Press.
Kay, D. W. K., & Burrows, G. D. (1984). *Handbook of studies on psychiatry and old age.* New York: Elsevier.
Levy, R., & Post, F. (1982). *The psychiatry of late life.* Boston: Blackwell Scientific Publications.
Pitt, B. (1974). *Psychogeriatrics: An introduction to the psychiatry of old age.* London: Churchill Livingstone.

7
Alzheimer's Disease and Related Disorders

Jeffrey R. Foster

I. Introduction

Critical issues concerning organic dimensions of geriatric psychopathology are encountered daily by psychiatrists. In this chapter, we will review some useful generalizations in approaching such disorders. We will illustrate these perspectives with case vignettes. Finally, we will more formally review categories of medical disturbances often associated with organic mental disorders in the elderly.

II. Approaches to Geriatric Organic Psychopathology

A. General Orientation
   1. Psychiatric diagnosis: If geriatric psychiatry is arbitrarily defined as encompassing diagnosis and treatment of disorders between the ages of 60 and 100, the field includes some 40% of the human lifespan. Correct diagnosis requires (1) an awareness of age-related normal changes in mental status across this lifespan; (2) knowledge of altered psychopathologic syndromes as aging progresses; (3) detection and assessment of several concurrent disturbances (e.g., depression plus cognitive impairment); and (4) appreciation of rapid changes that can occur in each of the psychiatric disturbances.
   2. Familiarity with medical illnesses that can affect mental status in older adults. This includes appreciation of medical disorders that can present predominantly with mental-status changes.

3. Familiarity with drugs (medical and psychiatric) that can adversely affect mental status and brain functioning. This includes awareness of age-related changes in pharmacokinetics and pharmacodynamics of individual drugs and their combined interactions.
4. Treatment Approaches
   a. Eliminate or reduce medications wherever possible.
   b. Stabilize medical conditions wherever possible.
   c. Carefully follow mental status and see if steps (a) and (b) ameliorate the psychiatric disturbances.
   d. Initiate immediate psychopharmacologic intervention for urgent disturbances (e.g., psychosis) only on a temporary basis while awaiting results of steps (a) and (b).
   e. Taper psychiatric medications as soon as possible to see if the disturbance has stabilized without need for their continuation.
   f. After an adequate trial on initial psychotropics, revise psychiatric drugs and psychotherapeutic approaches if the disturbances persist.
   g. Even though a patient may have an irreversible dementing illness, improvement of concurrent medical or psychiatric illnesses may substantially improve some aspects of cognitive functioning and improve quality of life for his or her remaining years.
   h. For patients with irreversible dementia, educational and psychotherapeutic emphases with the supporting family may alleviate stress and improve quality of life for everyone (Mace & Rabins, 1981).

B. Some Further Perspectives on Geriatric Organic Psychopathology
   1. Mental-status changes and behavioral disturbances in older adults do not necessarily reflect organic brain changes. Almost every major psychiatric disorder of adult life may present for the first time in the senescent years (e.g., major affective disorders; schizophrenia; paranoid states) (Foster & Reisberg, 1984).
   2. Any change in mental status showing a new or worsening degree of cognitive impairment (i.e., decrements in memory function and disorientation) should be regarded as abnormal and potentially reversible in cause.
   3. All mental-status and behavioral changes, regardless of cause, should be assumed to be potentially reversible (partly or completely) until proven otherwise. Thus comprehensive evaluation (medical, neurologic, and psychiatric) is indicated.
   4. The senescent brain is more sensitive to a variety of adverse physiologic and iatrogenic influences. Thus altered or impaired brain function is more frequent in the elderly and more likely to

reflect a diversity of systemic or focal disturbances or iatrogenic side effects. Examples of such brain disturbance would include excess sedation, confusion, dizziness, or gait difficulties (Salzman, 1984, pp. 4-6).
5. Older persons often have a concurrence of multiple medical illnesses and treatment regimens. These are often chronic in nature, with each illness capable of acute exacerbations or complications. Fluxes in each illness or their combination can produce mental-status abnormalities. Thus differential diagnosis (medical and psychiatric) is usually not an either-or proposition. Instead, it is a relative "sorting" of which disturbance or side effect is more operative (new or worsened) in affecting brain function (see "Vignettes" below).
6. Sometimes the correct identification and treatment of somatic causes does not relieve the mental-status abnormalities. In such cases, subsequent psychiatric treatment is needed. There appear to be two broad categories of such nonresponsiveness:
    a. Autonomous psychopathology, especially major affective disorders. An example would be a significant depression associated with either hyperthyroidism or hypothyroidism. Correction to a euthyroid state may not alleviate the depression, and antidepressant treatment will be required. It is as if the thyroid disturbance "triggered" the depression, which then took on an autonomous life of its own as a separate clinical entity.
    b. Cumulative psychopathology, especially cognitive impairment syndromes. An example would be a patient who suffers repeated episodes of delirium in which the sensorium clears after each episode; however, another bout of delirium leaves distinct cognitive impairment that persists, although the medical causes have been reversed. It is as if subclinical decrements have occurred over the delirious episodes and the last brain insult surpassed a cumulative threshold where the cognitive deficits become manifest, resulting in permanent impairment (Liston, 1982, pp. 61-62).
7. The brain is the source of mentation and behavior. The obviousness of this fact often becomes lost in the multiplicity of concurrent illnesses, drugs, treatment regimens, and cascade of laboratory data. The central position of brain functioning must be retained, since all diagnostic and treatment efforts are directed toward reversing altered status toward normal.

C. Many of the foregoing points are summarized in Figure 7.1.
   If we conceptualize geropsychiatric assessment as having several

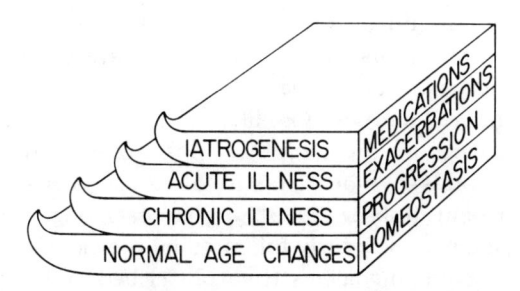

FIGURE 7.1 "Dissection" of geriatric psychopathology.

domains that must all be evaluated, the domains have a hierarchy of clinical priority.
1. First one considers iatrogenic factors, particularly medications, since these may be the quickest adverse influences to correct.
2. Next we attend to the issue of acute illness or acute exacerbations of chronic illness.
3. Then we assess the potential contributing role of chronic illness, which may be stable or subtly progressive.
4. Finally, we consider the influences of normal age-related changes, which evolve to different degrees over time in many organ systems but which together can progressively encroach on overall homeostatic integrity. All four domains frequently contribute to geriatric psychopathology, and their interactions give geropsychiatry a distinctive complexity, as illustrated in the following vignettes.

D. Vignettes. These three cases illustrate the occurrence of abnormal mental status in the context of multiple medical illnesses. In each instance the mental changes are likely due to the medical illnesses and/or drug side effects. The examples are not intended to reflect case management. Such cases are frequent, and their complexity contributes to the distinctiveness of geriatric psychiatry.
1. Case I: An elderly male patient with hypertensive cardiovascular disease currently presents with congestive heart failure and mild renal failure. He is on a sodium-restricted diet and takes the following prescribed medicines: digoxin, a diuretic, a potassium supplement, and an antihypertensive. A new physician recently added a "sleeping pill," due to nocturnal "restlessness." He also takes a laxative and two other unknown medicines he buys over-the-counter. Coincident with the initiation of the "sleeping pill" and increasing cardiac symptoms, he has become progressively

"confused" and unreliable in following his medical regimen. Pertinent mental-status findings show moderate cognitive impairment, whereas five days earlier he had a clear sensorium.
   a. Comment: The two most likely causes of his recent cognitive impairment are the congestive heart failure and the "sleeping pills." Congestive heart failure alone may cause such cerebral impairment (Libow, 1973). In like fashion, any CNS-acting medicine may be poorly tolerated by the elderly. The combination of eight medicines (five prescribed and three over-the-counter) is a common problem of polypharmacy among the elderly. The recent unreliability in adhering to his regimen raises the possibility that too many pills were taken, and this compounds the likelihood of drug side effects. Most cardiac and antihypertensive medicines have CNS effects and can cause alterations in mental status. Finally, unexplained or progressive "restlessness" in the elderly may be evidence of worsening mental status and requires a full diagnostic workup.
2. Case II: An elderly female with Parkinson's disease had a recent fall and complained of back pain. She struck her head but did not lose consciousness. The fall was believed to be due to worsening of her neurologic disease, and her Sinemet (levodopa plus carbidopa) was increased. She has a history of breast cancer; a mastectomy five years earlier had shown no evidence of metastases. Skull films are normal and spine films show no fracture, but a questionable luscent area is noted and possible metastatic disease is suggested. Shortly after the fall and Sinemet increase she suddenly had a first episode of visual hallucinations and paranoid delusions. She is alert, uncooperative, and mildly agitated. She refuses to answer many questions, and her orientation cannot be easily ascertained on the initial examination.
   a. Comment: The case illustrates altered mental status in the context of increased drug dose, head trauma, and possible metastatic disease. L-dopa is a CNS dopamine agonist and known to provoke psychotic states. Sequelae of head trauma could include a subdural hematoma, and a negative skull film does not exclude this possibility. Metastatic disease with systemic or direct cerebral involvement may produce altered mental status (Slaby & Wyatt, 1974). All elements need thorough evaluation.
3. Case III: A recently retired man has diabetes mellitus with peripheral vascular disease and cardiac complications. Gangrene of one leg is ascending, and an amputation is recommended. He has prided himself on his physical vigor, and the prospect of amputa-

tion leaves him depressed. He is eating and sleeping poorly but is cooperative and well oriented, with intact recent and remote memory. While awaiting surgery he develops congestive heart failure with arrhythmias that respond to treatment with two new medications. His blood glucose is well controlled, yet his mental status deteriorates, with clear emergence of disorientation and increasing anxiety. He is afebrile, but the gangrene is worsening; he is in pain, and another infection is becoming evident.

  a. Comment: Gangrene may produce nonspecific metabolic derangements affecting the cerebrum. Infectious processes may add to homeostatic imbalance and also contribute to cognitive dysfunction (Libow, 1973). The recent cardiac medications may be causing CNS side effects. The cognitive decline is superimposed on a substantial depression, and both the CNS dysfunction and the mood disturbance must be examined.

III. Etiology of Organic Psychopathology in Older Adults

Almost any illness occurring in adult life can present in the later years and affect brain function, with consequent abnormalities detected on mental-status examination. The psychiatric impairments may evolve abruptly or insidiously. Any list of causative diseases is incomplete, especially considering the frequent case in the elderly where multiple illnesses or drug side effects are concurrent. The following categories cover the more common disturbances encountered by the clinician. The list begins with direct brain structural effects and then moves to more systemic influences. The order chosen may be helpful for differential diagnostic thinking and does not reflect the frequency of the disorders (see Table 7.1).

TABLE 7.1 Frequent Causes of Organic Mental Disorders in the Elderly

Primary intracranial pathology	Secondary to extracranial systemic pathology
Trauma	Brain perfusion
CSF flow disturbance	Hypoxia/anoxia
Diffuse parenchymatous CNS disease	Toxic metabolic
	Hematologic
Tumor	Infectious
Vascular	Nutritional
	Febrile state

A. Trauma: subdural hematoma, cerebral concussion.
B. CSF flow disturbance: normal pressure hydrocephalus.
C. Diffuse parenchymatous CNS disease: Alzheimer's disease, Pick's disease, Parkinson's disease, Huntington's chorea, Creutzfeldt-Jacob disease, Wilson's disease, multiple sclerosis, sarcoidosis, other degenerative CNS diseases.
D. Brain tumor: meningeal, primary brain, vascular, metastatic, distal (nonmetastatic) effects of malignant neoplasia.
E. Vascular: multi-infarct dementia, arteriosclerosis, stroke, inflammatory blood vessel disease, arteriovenous malformations, collagen diseases, lacunar states, vertebral basilar insufficiency, transient ischemic episodes.
F. Brain perfusion: carotid artery disease, aortic arch syndrome, decreased cardiac output due to arrhythmia, congestive heart failure, pulmonary emboli, myocardial infarction, hypotension (especially systolic or orthostatic decreases due to psychiatric or other medications), hypovolemia, dehydration, GI bleeding.
G. Hypoxia and anoxia: cardiac arrest, anemia, chronic lung disease with hypoxia and/or hypercapnea, carbon monoxide poisoning.
H. Toxic-metabolic
   1. Medications: errors in self-administration, chlorpropamide (Diabinase) induced inappropriate ADH secretion leading to water intoxication, diuretic induced dehydration and electrolyte imbalance, drug-induced psychoses (e.g., L-dopa, indomethacin, steroids, etc.), all drugs with primary CNS-desired actions, drug toxicity (psychiatric medicines, Dilantin, digoxin, Inderal, antihypertensives, phenobarbital, etc.).
   2. Drug/alcohol abuse: bromides, barbiturates, alcohol encephalopathy, and so forth.
   3. Hypercalcemia: due to carcinoma, hyperparathyroidism, multiple myeloma, Paget's disease with immobilization, thiazide administration.
   4. Hyperglycemia: ketoacidosis, lactic acidosis, nonacidotic hyperosmolarity syndrome.
   5. Hypoglycemia: due to pancreatic insulinomas, exogenous insulin, sulfonylureas.
   6. Hypothyroidism.
   7. Hyperthyroidism: presenting with depression and/or apathy ("apathetic hyperthyroidism").
   8. Hypernatremia: hyperosmolar state due to inadequate fluid intake, cerebral concussion, excessive sweating with insufficient water intake, iatrogenic (e.g., hypertonic saline by IV or IP route, tube feeding of high-protein mixtures).

9. Hyponatremia: hypoosmolar syndrome due to increased ADH secretion, bronchogenic carcinoma, CVA, skull fracture, postoperative state, and so forth.
10. Azotemia: worsening of nephritis with UTI, medication-induced dehydration or hypokalemic nephropathy, obstructive uropathy, and so forth.
11. Hepatic failure: due to cirrhosis or hepatitis.
12. Adrenal: Addison's or Cushing's disease.

I. Hematologic: anemia, polycythemia, thrombocytosis, thrombocytopenia.
J. Infectious: cerebral abscess, TB, syphilis or gumma, encephalitis, other (bacterial, parasites, spirochetes, virus, fungal), subacute bacterial endocarditis.
K. Nutritional: thiamine, ascorbic acid, pellagra (niacin deficiency), B12 deficiency (pernicious anemia; may present with major mental changes), folate deficiency.
L. Any febrile condition.

REFERENCES

Foster, J. R., & Reisberg, B. (1984). Effects of aging on psychiatric disorders beginning earlier in life. In D. W. K. Kay & G. D. Burrows (Eds.), *Handbook of studies on psychiatry and old age* (pp. 265–276). New York: Elsevier.

Libow, L. S. (1973). Pseudosenility: Acute and reversible organic brain syndromes. *J Am Geriatric Society, 21,* 112–120.

Liston, E. H. (1982). Delirium in the aged. *Psychiatric Clinics of North America, 5*(1), 49–66.

Mace, N. L., & Rabins, P. V. (1981). *The 36-hour day.* Baltimore: Johns Hopkins University Press.

Salzman, C. (1984). *Clinical geriatric psychopharmacology.* New York: McGraw-Hill.

Slaby, A. E. S., & Wyatt, R. J. (1974). *Dementia in the presenium.* Springfield, IL: Charles C. Thomas.

ADDITIONAL READINGS

Eisdorfer, C., & Fann, W. E. (Eds.). (1982). *Treatment of psychopathology in the aging.* New York: Springer.

Jarvik, L. F., & Small, G. W. (Eds.). (1982). Aging [Special issue]. *Psychiatric Clinics of North America, 5*(1).

Kay, D. W. K., & Burrows, G. D. (1984). *Handbook of studies on psychiatry and old age.* New York: Elsevier.

Raskin, A., & Jarvik, L. F. (Eds.). (1979). *Psychiatric symptoms and cognitive loss in the elderly*. New York: Hemisphere Publishing.

Raskind, M. A., & Storrie, M. C. (1980). The organic mental disorders. In E. W. Busse & D. G. Blazer (Eds.), *Handbook of geriatric psychiatry* (pp. 305-328). New York: Van Nostrand Reinhold.

Reisberg, B. (1983). *Alzheimer's disease*. New York: The Free Press.

Sloan, R. B. (1980). Organic brain syndrome. In J. E. Birren & R. B. Sloane (Eds.), *Handbook of mental health and aging* (pp. 554-590). Englewood Cliffs, NJ: Prentice-Hall.

Wells, C. E. (Ed.). (1971). *Dementia*. Philadelphia: Davis.

8
Psychotherapy with the Elderly

Lawrence W. Lazarus and Joel Sadavoy

I. Introduction

In this chapter, we will discuss some of the developmental challenges of later life, barriers to engaging elderly patients in psychotherapy, issues discussed during therapy, various psychotherapeutic approaches (individual, family, group), and the results of recent outcome studies.

II. Developmental Challenges and Tasks of Later Life, Intrapsychic and Family

A. Intrapsychic (Atchley, 1982; Breslau, 1987; Cath, 1976; Erikson, 1968; Kohut, 1977; Meissner, 1975; Muslin & Epstein, 1980; Nemiroff & Colarusso, 1985; Sadavoy, 1987)
   1. Elderly persons attempt to find restitution and compensation for the inevitable biopsychosocial stresses and losses associated with the aging process. They struggle to maintain self-esteem, and a sense of purpose in life, during a phase of the life cycle sometimes characterized by diminishing ego resources and increasing narcissistic vulnerabilities and injuries. Potential losses include, but are not necessarily in the following order of importance to each elderly individual:
      a. Unmasked marital conflicts when children leave home.
      b. Retirement and fears of lost status.
      c. Reduced economic resources.
      d. A sense of disappointment in not realizing one's aspirations.
      e. Reduced sexual potency.

f. Loss of spouse and other relatives and friends through death or geographic relocation.
   g. Death of an adult child.
   h. Failing health.
   i. Illness and disability in one's spouse/significant others.
   j. Approaching death.
2. Authors have given a variety of perspectives on psychological issues in later life. Erikson (1968) conceptualized the last phase of life as characterized by the attainment of ego integrity or by failure to do so, resulting in a state of despair and disgust. Nemiroff and Colarusso (1985) stress the potential in later life for a continuation of psychological maturation and development.
3. Cath (1976) characterized the middle and later years as a balance between factors that promote a person's self-esteem and sense of self (e.g., wisdom derived from lifelong experience, the attainment of a satisfying philosophical and religious world view, past accomplishments, and the continuing opportunity for satisfaction of instinctual drives) versus factors leading to emotional depletion (e.g., failing health, cognitive impairment). Given adequate ego resources and a sustaining, supportive environment, most elderly people master the challenges of later life.
4. Atchley (1982) believes the elderly defend themselves against a negative self-image by:
   a. Focusing on past successes.
   b. Discounting messages that do not fit with their existing self-concept.
   c. Refusing to apply general beliefs and myths about aging to themselves.
   d. Chosing to interact with people who provide an egosyntonic experience.
   e. Perceiving selectively what they are told.
5. Persons who lose self-esteem in later life tend to do so because physical changes become so pronounced that they are forced to accept a less desirable self-image; because self-esteem had previously been too dependent on social or work roles; because they lost control over the environment to such an extent as to become essentially defenseless. While fear of death is widely discussed as a theoretical issue in aging, its clinical centrality is debatable. As a rule, the elderly, especially the very old, do not seem to fear death (Berezin, 1987; Pollock, 1987). Instead, they fear disability, pain, and dependency.
6. Traditional psychoanalytic theories of age-specific issues confronting the aged include:

a. Anxiety about disability and dependency.
   b. Neurotic defenses against castration anxieties.
   c. Attempts to exercise neurotic control over the environment by excluding psychologically painful stimuli (e.g., selectively hearing what one wants to hear).
   d. Apathy secondary to incapacity for affectionate relationships.
   e. Weakening of repressive barriers, with reduced capacity to tolerate regression. An additional phase-specific issue is seen in resistance to aging (i.e., resistance to accepting age-specific changes).
B. The Family (Benedek, 1970; Blenker, 1965; Sussman, 1965)
   1. Some of the developmental tasks for the elderly person regarding the family include:
      a. Accommodation to the role of grandparent and great-grandparent.
      b. Changing relationships with one's adult children.
      c. Adjustment to a spouse's increasing dependency and debility.
      d. Adjustment to widowhood.
      e. Acting as the repository and conveyer of family history and myths.
   2. Adult children of aging parents face developmental tasks that sometimes include:
      a. Assuming a parenting role with aging parents (e.g., providing emotional and financial support, physical care, and transportation).
      b. Mourning the death of a parent.
      c. Reactivation of old family conflicts, for example, sibling rivalry between the adult children for the parents' affections; family disagreement about who will assume the caregiver role; ambivalence about institutionalization; disputes about division of the family estate; and emotional overinvolvement or withdrawal. Sometimes adult children appear to totally reject their aging parents because of a history of parental abuse when the now-adult children were growing up or because the aging parents are perceived as evil, whether this is true or not.

III. Barriers to Psychotherapy
(Butler & Lewis, 1973; Gaitz, 1974; Lazarus & Weinberg, 1980)

A. These can be divided into barriers related to patient, family, physician, and society.

1. Patient-Related Barriers
   a. Some elderly people believe that unhappiness, depression, and anxiety are expected concomitants of the later years and attribute these abnormal psychological states to physical causes, thus seeking out medical, and avoiding psychiatric, treatment.
   b. Some are deterred from psychiatric treatment because they were raised in an era when shame and embarrassment were associated with such treatment or because of local attitudinal beliefs about psychiatry common to their geographic locale.
   c. The psychiatric symptoms themselves (e.g., hopelessness, apathy, cognitive impairment).
   d. Such practical deterrents as cost (e.g., Medicare limitations) and transportation problems.
2. Family-Related Barriers
   a. Adult children of aging parents may minimize and attribute psychiatric symptoms to "growing old."
   b. The family may hesitate suggesting psychiatric assessment to an aging family member because of ambivalence about assuming a parenting, caregiving role and fear of the aging member's disapproval and anger.
   c. The family's need to maintain an idealized image of the family member.
   d. Conscious or unconscious ambivalence and resentment toward the aging parent, preventing needed medical and psychiatric intervention.
   e. Negative, stereotypic family attitudes toward psychiatry.
3. Physician-Related Barriers (Karasu & Waltzman, 1972)
   a. Adoption of negative, prejudicial attitudes toward the elderly; for example, the belief that a shortened life expectancy renders the elderly unsuitable for psychotherapy.
   b. Countertransference reactions to elderly patients.
   c. Concern with patient disapproval if referral is made to a psychiatrist.
   d. Frustration and therapeutic nihilism when faced with chronic illness, dying, and death.
4. Societal and Health Care System–Related Barriers
   a. Inadequate Medicare and other third-party reimbursement for outpatient psychotherapy.
   b. The traditional biomedical model of health care has tended to espouse a medical orientation to the elderly, with comparatively less importance placed on psychosocial and behavioral aspects of illness and treatment.

IV. Establishing the Therapeutic Relationship
(Butler & Lewis, 1973; Goldfarb, 1956; Kahana, 1979; Lazarus & Weinberg, 1980; Meerloo, 1961; Pfeiffer, 1971; Yesavage & Karasu, 1982)

A. Because of the complexity of symptom presentation and the rapidly changing clinical course, the therapist needs to maintain considerable flexibility when selecting and utilizing various therapeutic modalities.
  1. The therapist may assume different roles at different points in time with the same patient, such as that of a primary-care physician, psychopharmacologist, individual or family therapist, and member of a health care team.
  2. At the beginning of an initial interview with a somatically oriented patient, a medically oriented interview style may feel more comfortable and familiar to the patient.
  3. The initial visit may require more than one hour because of the patient's complex and extensive personal and family history.
  4. The "identified" elderly patient is usually interviewed first and alone. That approach denotes respect for the patient and may elicit information not otherwise obtainable. It is informative and facilitates the therapeutic alliance if family members are also interviewed. Not only may other family members, or the entire family, require treatment, but vital information may be obtained from them when interviewed both in the absence and the presence of the elderly patient.
  5. The therapist's stance is usually active when obtaining information and working through patient and family resistances to therapy.
  6. Patients may require the therapist to speak slowly, loudly, and concretely and to demonstrate (by word and sometimes by touch) concern, respect, and realistic hopefulness.
  7. Since depressed patients often feel hopeless about obtaining anything from the therapist, it is useful to demonstrate an active willingness to help.
  8. Patients need to feel that they have obtained help from the first interview (e.g., the therapist's empathic response to the patient's predicament, medication, and/or active intervention in an aspect of the patient's life).
  9. Some patients solicit the therapist's approval and affirmation that they are not "crazy" in an attempt to restore self-esteem and allay fears about talking to a psychiatrist.

10. To facilitate compliance and cooperation, the treatment plan is individualized and explained in terms that the patient and family can understand.
11. Treatment goals realistically consider the patient's limitations in order to avoid frustration and a sense of failure.
12. The therapist needs to coordinate treatment with other health professionals involved in the patient's care.

V. Individual Psychotherapy

A. Goals (Gotestam, 1980; Kahana, 1979; Nemiroff & Colarusso, 1985; Pollock, 1987; Yesavage & Karasu, 1982).
   1. For the aged, in contrast to younger patients, goals should be more focused and stated explicitly. Goals may include:
      a. Improvement of interpersonal relationships.
      b. Enhancement of productivity and achievement of life satisfaction.
      c. Helping patients to actualize their current potential and enhance their sense of completeness and dignity.
      d. Psychological mastery over the past as a basis for current adaptation.
      e. Helping patients come to terms with conflicts and anxieties over mortality and death.
      f. Relief of suffering.
      g. Appropriate acceptance of dependency.
      h. Improving the patient's ability to utilize caregivers and community resources.
      i. Establishing a therapeutic relationship to aid adaptation to, and restitution of, the losses of aging.
   2. Additional goals for patients able to undertake more intensive, psychoanalytically oriented psychotherapy aimed at structural or intrapsychic change may include:
      a. Reawakening of suppressed passions, rages, and old allegiances, which may have become psychologically unacceptable, or experienced as useless to the aging individual.
      b. Mourning of that which has passed.
      c. Resolving interpersonal conflicts, often stemming from the past, which are now emotionally draining.
      d. Working through of intensely private, conflicted, and shame-engendering past experiences.
      e. Establishing a transference and working through conflicts in the transference.

3. For the frail elderly, goals are more limited and include using psychotherapeutic understanding to aid in:
    a. Adapting the environment to the needs of the patient, rather than the reverse.
    b. Strengthening the roles of the caregivers, such as the family or the institution.
    c. Sometimes a limited mourning process may be encouraged, keeping in mind the patient's psychological limitations.

B. Indications for Individual Psychotherapy (Berezin, 1987; Blau & Berezin, 1975; Kahana, 1979, 1987; Lazarus & Weinberg, 1980; Nemiroff & Colarusso, 1985; Pollock, 1982, 1987; Rechtschaffen, 1959).
    1. While persons over the age of 65 constitute 10% of the population, they make up only 2-4% of the psychiatric outpatient population, despite the finding that 25% of them have anxiety, depression, and other disorders. Advanced age per se is not a contraindication to psychotherapy; indeed, the efficacy of psychotherapy with the elderly has been repeatedly demonstrated (Rechtschaffen, 1959). The improved educational level of increasing numbers of aged persons and greater societal acceptance of psychotherapy is slowly leading to more self-referrals.
    2. From a psychotherapeutic perspective, the aged can be grouped as follows:
        a. The aging group—characterized by noncrippling physical change or illness; conflicts over self-expression and actual accomplishments versus aspirations; retirement issues; fluctuation of instinctual drives; awareness of time limitations and mortality; loss of significant others; and changing marital, parental, and occupational relationships.
        b. The crisis group—characterized by sudden major loss, work failures, or interpersonal crises.
        c. The frail, debilitated group—characterized by chronic, debilitating illnesses; brain damage; constricted activity; need for assistance in activities of daily living; regressive behavior; lost sources of external gratification; and increased vulnerability to grief reactions.
    3. The likeliest candidates for insight-oriented therapy are drawn from group 2a. Insight-oriented therapy is indicated when the patient needs to resolve a psychodynamically determined issue (e.g., dependency or grief) that is causing psychiatric symptoms. Impaired capacity to resolve grief and mourning is an example

of a specific indication for psychotherapy. Favorable prognostic indicators of insight-oriented therapy include:
  a. Motivation for change.
  b. Capacity to utilize insight, form and resolve transference.
  c. Capacity for self-observation.
  d. Ability to mourn.
  e. Previous capacity for work and pleasure.
  f. Ability to tolerate painful affects.
4. In general, supportive psychotherapy and crisis intervention are more appropriate for groups 2b and 2c, although crisis intervention may evolve into longer-term, insight-oriented therapy. However, if the patient does not possess the potential resources for new and adaptive behavior, it is wise not to tamper with necessary psychological defenses unless substitutes can be offered, for example, new sustaining relationships or supportive environmental changes. This caution is especially relevant to the severely ill or otherwise severely disadvantaged patient (Muslin & Epstein, 1980).
5. Psychotherapy for the frail elderly generally does not aim at conflict resolution. Instead, therapists use their psychodynamic understanding to help patients increase their realistic tolerance for incapacities and to explore means to ameliorate problems through environmental change (Yesavage & Karasu, 1982). These patients are often institutionalized, cognitively impaired, and rarely self-referred (Goldfarb, 1956).

C. Age-specific Issues in Psychotherapy
  1. Transference (Blau & Berezin, 1975; Gotestam, 1980; Grunes, 1987; King, 1980; Nemiroff & Colarusso, 1985).
     a. Transference is unconscious, not time-bound, and does not follow chronological calendar considerations. Hence age-specific transferences are debatable. Developmental theory suggests that transference in the aging individual is multigenerational in origin, reflecting not only childhood experience, but also real relationships established during adulthood as well.
     b. Transference manifestations include:
        (1) Reverse transference as coined by Grunes (1987)—the therapist becomes the child of the patient, whom the patient may experience as the guarantor of his immortality.
        (2) Parental transferences.
        (3) Erotic (lover-spouse) transference, which may help the working through of mourning for lost opportunities, youth, and sexuality.

(4) Other key figures of adult life (confidant, spouse, close colleague, sibling).
  c. In the transference, regardless of the therapist's age, patients often experience themselves as small and helpless and the therapist as older and more powerful. The patient may therefore function on many time-scales during therapy. King (1980) suggests that conflicts ordinarily associated with adolescence may be especially important factors in later-life transferences. The patient reexperiences these conflicts, but with a reversed focus. These conflicts include sexual and biological losses; role changes and disengagements; dependency fears; changing from a two-generational to a one-generational home; need to make new relationships; and identity crisis secondary to breakdown of old defenses.
  d. Idealization of and use of the therapist as a parental surrogate is common, especially in institutionalized patients. It may stem from a projection of the patient's own grandiosity and unconscious need for a magical protector against fears associated with aging. Negative transference responses include viewing the therapist as an unwanted, uninvited helper, as an intrusive voyeur, or as a potential further source of rejection.
2. Countertransference (Cohen, 1982; Grunes, 1987; King, 1980; Lazarus & Weinberg, 1980; Nemiroff & Colarusso, 1985; Yesavage & Karasu, 1982)
  a. Therapists' countertransference may be responsible for the tendency to avoid treating the elderly. For some therapists, the elderly patient:
    (1) May at first appear unattractive or unproductive.
    (2) May be perceived as close to death and not warranting the therapist's efforts.
  b. The therapist may respond by:
    (1) Withdrawing from the task.
    (2) Being overzealous and feeling omnipotent.
    (3) Feeling diminished self-esteem and competency, especially when working with the chronically ill and dying patient.
  c. Countertransference reactions may also lead to greater self-awareness in the therapist and, for example, to constructive working through of relationships with the therapist's own parents and grandparents.
  d. Countertransference reactions to treating the aged include:
    (1) Mobilization of the therapist's fears of illness, decline, mortality, and death.

(2) Erotic countertransference—inexperienced therapists may be shocked at the development of a sexual transference. A belief in the asexuality of the aged may be a defense against unresolved conflicts over parental sexuality. Therapists may also have to cope with loss of the sexually desired parental object, who is no longer sexually attractive.
(3) Mobilized unresolved guilt toward the therapist's own parents.
(4) Fears of engulfment secondary to fear of the patient's helplessness and dependence, leading to rejection of the patient.
(5) Unconscious wishes to dominate the parent, leading to overcontrolling behavior in therapy.
(6) Idealization of the older patient, leading to unrealistic expectations of capacities and strengths.
(7) Unconscious wishes to be the favorite child.
(8) Grandiose need to conquer forces of aging.
(9) Unreasonable anger at the patient, perhaps secondary to the patient's regressive behavior.
(10) Overidentification, leading to pity and sadness, and blocking of the therapist's accurate empathy and realistic exploration of possibilities for change.
(11) Fear of termination—therapists may feel they are keeping their patients alive, and continued therapy becomes a defense to ward off concerns over the patients' death.
(12) Unconscious avoidance of empathizing with the patient's intense loneliness and loss.
(13) Unconscious hostility to the therapist's own parents may lead to watering down the therapeutic process by inappropriately relying on supportive, covering techniques and avoiding deeper areas of psychological conflict.

3. Expressions of Resistance (Breslau, 1987; King, 1980; Lewis & Butler, 1974; Sadavoy, 1987)
   a. Similar expressions of resistance occur in the elderly as in the younger adult patient but with different emphasis; for example, in the elderly there is a decrease in dramatic forms of acting-out. Aging may actually reduce resistance in some ways. For example, the patient may have less difficulty integrating interpretations.
   b. Manifestations of resistance include:
      (1) Denial of aging; for example, through inappropriate overactivity or youthful dress.

(2) Regression to more primitive defensive states, with overuse of projection, denial, splitting, and magical thinking.
(3) Withdrawal—especially as seen in institutions.
(4) Overreliance on reminiscence and the past.
(5) Inappropriate dependency or apparent confusion, pseudofragility or feigning deafness.
(6) Greater use of manipulation to replace formerly used, but now less useful, defenses such as sexuality or social status.
(7) Avoidance of therapy with claims of illness or immobility in order to avoid appearing stupid or crazy.

D. Process of Therapy (Blau & Berezin, 1975; Goldfarb, 1956; Grunes, 1987; Kahana, 1979; Pollock, 1987; Sadavoy, 1987; Yesavage & Karasu, 1982)
  1. General Principles
     a. Therapy may occur in a variety of settings, including:
        (1) Office.
        (2) Institution.
        (3) Patient's home.
     b. Basic guidelines for therapy include:
        (1) Using the least disruptive interventions when dealing with crises.
        (2) If not done previously, an initial, thorough medical workup is important to rule out physical illness as a cause for psychiatric symptomatology.
        (3) Mobilization of family and community resources may be necessary.
        (4) Using medications judiciously in conjunction with psychotherapy.
        (5) Avoidance of stereotypic responses and generalized rules.
        (6) Formation of an accurately empathic relationship.
        (7) The therapist may act as a real or symbolic replacement for the patient's losses.
        (8) The therapist should be prepared for a possible long-term therapy commitment.
        (9) Monitoring of the patient for ongoing deterioration during the course of therapy and adapting techniques as necessary. For example, emotionally charged discussions will often need to be titrated in keeping with the patient's tolerance, or the time, duration, and frequency of sessions changed.
  2. Techniques of Psychotherapy (Kahana, 1979; Yesavage & Karasu, 1982)—these may be divided into three main categories,

depending on the capacities and the support network of the particular patient.
   a. Insight promotion. Therapy is intermediate to long-term. In general the most frequently used techniques include:
      (1) Clarification (preconscious to conscious awareness).
      (2) Interpretation (unconscious to conscious awareness).
      (3) Promotion and utilization of the transference. Therapy most often occurs in the office setting, where 45-minute to 1-hour sessions occur at intervals ranging from once to five times a week. Therapy may continue for months or years.
   b. Adaptive intervention—especially indicated for crisis intervention and for the medically ill. The duration of therapy may be brief (from a few sessions to several weeks), at intervals from once to several times weekly. Techniques include support of the patient's healthier defenses and previous adaptive methods to reestablish the previous level of functioning without expecting major psychological reorganization.
   c. Basic support. Sessions vary in frequency, duration, and regularity—once a month is a common interval after the initial meetings. Therapy is based on the patient's conscious and unconscious needs and conflicts, which determine the supportive therapeutic stance; for example:
      (1) Reassurance (maternal or paternal stance).
      (2) Narcissistic support (e.g., mirroring stance).
      (3) Therapist reinforcing the patient's perception of him or her as a magical savior.
      (4) Therapist as a manager (medical or parental stance).
   d. Other supportive techniques include ventilation and reminiscence. Especially for debilitated elderly patients, environmental manipulation is necessary (e.g., a comforting bedtime routine). Caregivers are often given advice and education. Therapy is less exploratory of taboo subjects and less metaphorical. It is more concrete and information-giving, active, structured, and slower paced, with implicit acknowledgment of the patient's limitations (Lawton, 1976).
3. Stage of Psychotherapy (Gotestam, 1980; Grunes, 1987; Lazarus & Weinberg, 1980; Nemiroff & Colarusso, 1985)
   a. Opening phase—this phase is referred to in IV on page 151.
   b. Middle (working-through) phase (Kahana, 1979; Myers, 1984; Nemiroff & Colarusso, 1985)—this phase is reached only in selected cases. Transference develops, evolves, and is open to interpretation. Dream analysis is possible. Despite life issues and themes related to aging, the process is similar

to treatment of younger patients. The reader is referred to detailed case studies in the literature (Nemiroff & Colarusso, 1985; Myers, 1984; Kahana, 1979).
   c. Termination (Cath, 1962; Nemiroff & Colarusso, 1985; Lazarus & Weinberg, 1980; Myers, 1984; Yesavage & Karasu, 1982)—the therapist indicates ongoing availability after the conclusion of therapy, since subsequent losses and conflicts are almost inevitable. Termination may reactivate the issues that initially led to treatment, fear about losing the therapist, as well as death anxieties. The patient may discuss disappointment about not having attained some lifelong goals and dreams. While positive aspects of the real and transference relationship, such as the patient's sense of security and caring from the therapist, may be hard to relinquish because they fill a void of loneliness, many elderly have other important relationships and can tolerate termination.

VI. Specialized Individual Psychotherapy Techniques

A. Reminiscence, or Life-Review Therapy (Lewis & Butler, 1974)
   1. Life-review is a universal mental process, initiated by the realization of mortality and characterized by the progressive return of memories of past experiences, especially those that were conflictual. The purpose of life review therapy is to enhance reminiscence and make it more conscious and deliberate. This technique is reported to resolve old problems; increase tolerance of conflict; relieve guilt and fears; and enhance creativity, generosity, and acceptance of the present.
   2. Life-review is facilitated by:
      a. Written or taped autobiographies.
      b. Pilgrimages to places of earlier experiences.
      c. Reunions.
      d. Genealogies.
      e. Memorabilia (scrapbooks, albums).
      f. Verbal or written summation of life's work.
      g. Promotion of ethnic identity.
   3. This therapeutic approach may be contraindicated for patients who have realistic guilt about the past or who are overwhelmed by unmourned or unresolved past disappointments and losses.
B. Brief Psychodynamic Therapy (Lazarus & Groves, 1987; Lewis & Butler, 1974)
   1. Brief, time-limited psychotherapy may be especially useful for the aged because of their shorter remaining lifespan, reduction

of dependency fears (of patient and therapist), more rapid pace, clearer circumscribed therapeutic focus, reduced costs, and the expectation that problems can be resolved.
  2. Most evident changes in brief psychodynamic therapy appear to be in the areas of symptomatic improvement and resolution of the focal problem, with comparatively less improvement in insight and self-understanding. Self-esteem is restored, and a positive self-image is often reestablished.
C. Psychotherapy in Institutions (Breslau, 1987; Goldfarb, 1956; Sadavoy, 1987; Sadavoy & Dorian, 1983)
  1. Goldfarb's (1956) technique—a special therapeutic technique for institutionalized elderly, many of whom have cognitive impairment and/or have suffered major losses. For these severely impaired patients, Goldfarb advocated that the therapist foster an illusion of being strong and omnipotent. By gratifying some of the patient's requests, the patient is encouraged to feel control and mastery over the therapist, thereby enhancing self-esteem. Sessions are brief—15 minutes once a week.
  2. Interdisciplinary team approach—goals of therapy include:
     a. Containing and limiting pathological behavior.
     b. Establishing a therapeutic alliance between patient, family, and the institution's staff.
     c. Developing a cohesive team approach to patient care.
     d. Reducing patient's psychological reliance on pathological symptoms.
     e. Methods include:
        (1) Diagnosis of environmental, interactional, and intrapsychic stressors and precipitants, including identifying behavioral interactions promoting aberrant behaviors.
        (2) Establishing a written, itemized treatment plan that includes, from the outset, the collaboration of staff, patient, and family.
        (3) Weekly staff education meetings that are focused on the psychological causes of the behaviors.
        (4) Individual psychotherapy with the patient when possible, and counseling the family in order to develop specific understanding of, and constructive responses to, the patient's behavior.
D. Cognitive Therapy (Beck, Rush, Shaw, & Emery, 1979; Karasu, 1986; Thompson, Gallagher, & Breckenridge, 1987)
  1. Cognitive therapy is a brief psychotherapy approach that attempts to correct the depressed patient's dysfunctional atti-

tudes and stereotyped self-defeating patterns of thought, and to promote integration of positive perceptions, thinking patterns, and self-awareness by utilizing interpretations, explanations, practical information, and/or direct confrontation.
2. The cognitive therapy model postulates three specific concepts to explain depression (Beck et al., 1979):
   a. The negative triad—an interactive set of negative views of oneself, the world, and the future. Depressed patients view themselves as deficient, the world as presenting insurmountable obstacles, and the future as a continuation of current difficulties.
   b. Underlying beliefs or schemata—negative perceptions and views precipitate changes in mood, leading to more negative thinking and hence more depression.
   c. Cognitive errors—the thinking pattern of depressed patients is typically distorted in the following ways:
      (1) Stylistically—tends to exaggerate the negatives and minimize the positives.
      (2) Semantically—inexact labeling of events, leading to personalization and affective overreaction.
      (3) Formally—thinking patterns tend to be automatic and involuntary despite disconfirming evidence.
3. Aim of therapy—patients learn to reverse their negative cognitive sets by the following five processes:
   a. Learning to monitor negative thoughts.
   b. Recognizing connections between negative thoughts and feelings of depression.
   c. Examining the evidence for and against specific automatic thoughts.
   d. Learning to identify and alter dysfunctional beliefs that sustain these negative cognitions.
   e. Developing more reality-oriented or adaptive views of themselves, the world, and the future.
4. Common cognitive distortions in the elderly (Gallagher & Thompson, 1982a)—it is especially important for the therapist to confront these distortions repeatedly, beginning in the early stages of therapy.
   a. "I'm too old to change." The therapist may say, "Perhaps it is true that you cannot learn new ways of thinking about your problems, but how will you know this for certain unless you try?"
   b. "If only my external situation would change, then I wouldn't

be depressed." The therapist may say, "It is more effective to attempt to change your view of the problem and to examine how your views contribute to depression."
   c. "You're too young to help me." The therapist questions the basic premise and encourages temporary suspension of this belief so that therapy can proceed.
5. Modification of cognitive therapy for the elderly (Gallagher & Thompson, 1982a)—some of these modifications are applicable to younger patients as well, but they warrant reviewing.
   a. Socialization into therapy by:
      (1) Eliciting the patient's expectations of therapy and presenting therapy as a way to learn to adjust better to this phase of the life cycle.
      (2) Explaining what cognitive therapy can and cannot do.
      (3) Emphasizing that cognitive therapy requires the patient's active participation.
   b. Enhancing learning capabilities by:
      (1) Presenting material in various ways (e.g., encourage patients to record notes in a therapy journal and to review the tape of each therapy session prior to the next session).
      (2) Using relevant, age-specific examples (e.g., perceptions about retirement, age-related bodily changes).
      (3) Encouraging the practice of cognitive therapy techniques outside therapy sessions.
      (4) Demonstrating understanding and patience for elderly patients who may be hesitant to follow through with homework assignments and to try new ways of thinking.
   c. Terminating therapy by:
      (1) Tapering off, rather than abruptly terminating, therapy.
      (2) Reviewing what has been learned and rehearsing for problems arising after treatment ends, using the newly learned cognitive skills.
      (3) Leaving the door open to return to therapy without shame or a sense of failure.
6. Indications for cognitive therapy—the limited number of controlled clinical studies indicate that this treatment may be suitable for elderly patients with:
   a. Dysthymic disorder.
   b. Major depression (especially acute nonpsychotic depressions with minimal endogenous features).

c. Motivation and the cognitive ability to try this approach.
7. Contraindications
   a. Significant cognitive impairment.
   b. Bipolar depressions and schizo-affective disorders.
   c. Schizophrenia.
8. Recent outcome studies (Gallagher, Thompson, & Breckenridge, 1987; Gallagher & Thompson, 1982b)—91 elderly patients with major depression were randomly assigned to one of the following three brief psychotherapies—cognitive, behavioral, or psychodynamic (16–20 individual sessions each). Results were:
   a. The overall positive response rate for the three therapies was 70% (52% had complete remission; 18% showed significant symptomatic improvement).
   b. All three therapies were equally effective. This result is similar to that obtained in a study of two types of group therapy with depressed elderly outpatients (Steuer et al., 1984), in which equally positive outcomes were found for cognitive/behavioral and psychodynamically oriented supportive-expressive approaches.
   c. Nonresponders to the three therapy modalities were characterized by:
      (1) Presence of endogenous signs.
      (2) Presence of a concomitant personality disorder.
      (3) Low patient expectation of a positive outcome.
   d. Follow-up assessments after completion of therapy showed a trend (not statistically significant) for patients treated with cognitive and behavioral therapy to maintain their improvement more than patients treated with psychodynamic therapy.
   e. Neither age per se nor sex was a predictor of outcome. Very elderly patients responded as well as the less elderly patients to the three treatment modalities.
9. An appraisal of cognitive therapy (Karasu, 1986)—positive aspects of cognitive therapy for adult and elderly patients include:
   a. Time-limited nature, reinforcing the expectation of positive change within a circumscribed period of time.
   b. Consideration of the elderly patient's limited financial resources.
   c. Support of higher-level defense mechanisms, such as intellectualization and rationalization.
   d. Encouragement of the patient's active participation.

e. Well-articulated, structured procedures for treatment of depression.
f. Potential for integration with other treatment modalities (e.g., behavioral, psychodynamic).
10. Some potential shortcomings include:
    a. Restricted application to depression and less severely impaired patients.
    b. Potential, when used as the sole treatment modality, to produce overintellectualization or mechanical application to fend off feelings.

E. Group Therapy (Burnside, 1984; Hartford, 1980; Leszcz, 1987; Leszcz, Feigenbaum, Sadavoy, & Robinson, 1985)
   1. Purposes include:
      a. Socialization.
      b. Enhancing attitudinal changes.
      c. Personal development (e.g., countering myths of aging and societal stereotypes).
      d. Learning and education.
      e. Behavioral change using behavior modification, reality orientation, and reality therapy.
      f. Emotional catharsis and life review.
      g. Problem solving.
      h. Bridge between the institution and the community.
   2. Composition—may vary, may be open or closed. In institutions, because of the predominance of women, men may benefit from a homogeneous male group; group size varies from 40 to the more common 5 to 8 patients.
   3. Goals—vary with composition, purpose, and setting. They complement and overlap goals of other therapies. Goals in institutions include:
      a. Halting regression.
      b. Resocialization.
      c. Reengagement.
      d. Problem solving.
      e. Information exchange.
   4. More general goals include:
      a. Enhancing self-esteem and hopefulness.
      b. Identification with therapists as role models.
      c. Opportunity for patients to give to and help others.
      d. Diagnostic clarification.
      e. Functional evaluation.
      f. Clarification and resolution of intrapsychic conflict.
      g. Provision of narcissistic supplies and restitution for losses.

h. Creating a safe forum for grief work.
i. Support through periods of crisis.
5. Leadership—a co-therapy relationship is often useful, especially a male-female therapy team, because it:
   a. Helps reduce stress on a single leader who must cope with such issues as the patients' dependency and group attrition through illness and death.
   b. Enhances role modeling.
   c. Enables the group to continue despite a leader's absence.
6. Group leadership styles vary, including:
   a. Facilitators.
   b. Managers.
   c. Advisors.
   d. Reinforcers.
   e. Clarifiers.
7. Inexperienced or untrained leaders require close supervision.
8. Themes and issues—echo those of individual treatment. Experienced group leaders have noted that death of group members seems well tolerated, with sadness but rarely anxiety. Loss of significant family members, friends, and personal capacities are central issues. In institutions, issues include:
   a. Staff-patient interactions.
   b. Environmental concerns.
   c. Patient interactions with each other and their families.
9. Affective themes surround issues of:
   a. Abandonment.
   b. Dependency.
   c. Pain and illness.
10. Altruistic or narcissistic themes arise around issues of:
    a. Closeness.
    b. Giving to and helping others.
11. Techniques—types of groups are dependent on the types of patients, the setting, and the leader's therapeutic orientation. Examples include:
    a. Psychoanalytically oriented psychotherapy.
    b. Activity.
    c. Rehabilitation.
    d. Music.
    e. Dance.
    f. Movement.
    g. Art.
    h. Dramatics.
    i. Writing.

j. Oral history.
k. Family.
l. Reminiscence.
m. Cognitive.
n. Behavioral.
o. Relaxation.
p. Meditation.
12. In psychodynamically oriented groups, the process first deals with group formation and cohesion with emphasis on the importance of regular attendance, focusing on enhancing safety for the individuals and on the group's integrity. Leadership is often active and directive, combining a focus on the "here and now" with reminiscing and using appropriate confrontations or interpretations of behavior, maladaptive defenses, and transference issues. Structured go-rounds, humor, life-review, and other exercises facilitate interpersonal awareness. Special attention is paid to the patients' fear of, and sensitivity to, devaluation or exclusion.
13. Regardless of the type of group, transference issues are evident. These issues include:
    a. Projection of idealized or ambivalent feelings onto the group leaders.
    b. Reactivation of early family conflicts, such as sibling rivalry. In some groups (e.g., task-oriented) these issues may be noted but dealt with instrumentally (e.g., separating conflicting members). Even in more verbally oriented groups, these issues are often dealt with in the "here and now," rather than responded to with genetic interpretations.
F. Family Therapy (Breslau, 1987; McEwan, 1987; Nagy & Spark, 1973; Ripeckyj & Lazarus, 1984; Sadavoy, 1987; Sadavoy & Dorian, 1983; Shanas, 1984): There is a relative paucity of research in this area despite the strong involvement of families with their elderly. Eight percent of American households are three-generational, and 82% of the elderly live within 30 minutes of at least one child.
1. Family assessment is an important part of every complete geropsychiatric workup, for purposes of gathering history and confirming data about the family system and creating a family treatment alliance that can facilitate, when necessary, further family therapy. Assessment generally involves evaluating stresses and strengths of a three- or more generational system. Four- and five-generation families are becoming more prevalent. Causes of stress within families include:

a. The adult child's denial of the aging parent's decline.
   b. Guilt and ambivalence over the burden of care.
   c. Enmeshment of caregivers with the patient.
   d. Guilt over institutionalization.
2. Nagy and Spark (1973) have classified the four generational roots of family stress:
   a. Loyalty—conflict over parent's expectation versus child's performance; uncertainty in the parent, the child, and/or the grandchild about the extent of the obligations imposed by loyalty to the aging family member.
   b. Entitlement and ledger-balancing—conflicts over verbal and nonverbal expectations of repayment, usually involving repayment by the child to the aging parent for the parent's past effort. The adult child is often in conflict over the right to put self-interest ahead of the parent's interest—for example, the daughter who jeopardizes her marriage because she cannot refuse her mother's demands for time, care, and attention.
   c. Justice—how much is enough and fair?
   d. Legacy for posterity—events, conflicts, and emotions are passed to succeeding generations and may lead to a legacy of health, justice, and fulfillment, or despair, disruption, jealousy, and betrayal—for example, a son's guilt at experiencing success and happiness in the face of his father's unspoken demand that he renounce pleasure as his father had been forced to do earlier in life.
3. Assessment takes into account:
   a. Diagnostic issues regarding individual family members.
   b. Crisis evaluation.
   c. Practical structural issues and problem solving.
   d. Affectional patterns.
   e. Family hierarchy and roles.
   f. Intrapsychic factors—especially in institutional settings, families are often scapegoated by the staff, who may assume the family is rejecting or too overinvolved with the patient.
4. Indications for family therapy include:
   a. Family education.
   b. Facilitation of anticipatory mourning.
   c. Management of inappropriate dependency relationships.
   d. Family-patient-staff institutional conflicts.
   e. Resolution of old family conflicts rekindled by stresses imposed by an aging family member's decline.
   f. Crisis resolution, for example, as caused by remarriages, or conflicts over finances and competency.

5. Techniques of therapy—the composition of family members and the focus of therapy can vary considerably. The treatment group may include:
   a. Three or more generations in a group.
   b. Selected subgroup (e.g., children only).
   c. Marital subgroup (e.g., aging couple).
   d. Child-grandchildren-great-grandchildren.
   e. Individual family member (but with a family focus).
6. Role of the Family Therapist
   a. Clarify issues and educate family about behavior and motivation of the aging family member as well as other family members.
   b. Advise on new techniques of behavior and problem solving.
   c. Where appropriate, elucidate and interpret unconscious conflicts.
   d. Help make realistic decisions and include the aging member in the process.
   e. Facilitate adaptation to institutionalization.
   f. Remain available to the family in the future.

VII. Summary

In summary, factors that distinguish psychotherapy with the elderly from that with younger adults include the discussions about late-life developmental tasks and challenges, formidable barriers and resistances to treatment, and the variety of transference and countertransference reactions that occur during therapy. The therapist understands that the patient's changing clinical needs may necessitate different forms of therapeutic interaction at different stages of therapy. The therapist is usually very active in working through patient and family resistances to therapy. Treatment goals are realistically tailored to the patient's current capabilities to avoid mutual frustration and disappointment. Most elderly patients seen by psychiatrists require more supportive forms of therapy, requiring the therapist to be active, directive, and involved with the patient in a real and meaningful way. Clinical reports and available outcome studies to date support the contention that elderly patients are very responsive to psychotherapy.

REFERENCES

Atchley, R. C. (1982). The aging self. *Psychotherapy: Theory, Research and Practice, 19,* 388-396.

Beck, A. T., Rush, A. J., Shaw, B. F., & Emery, G. (1979). *Cognitive therapy of depression.* New York: Guilford.

Benedek, T. (1970). Parenthood during the life cycle. In E. J. Antony (Ed.), *Parenthood* (pp. 185-206). Boston: Little, Brown.

Berezin, M. A. (1987). Reflections on psychotherapy with the elderly. In J. Sadavoy & M. Leszcz (Eds.), *Treating the elderly with psychotherapy: The scope for change in later life* (pp. 45-63). Madison, CT: International Universities Press.

Blau, D., & Berezin, M. A. (1975). Neuroses and character disorders. In J. G. Howells (Ed.), *Modern perspectives in the psychiatry of old age* (pp. 201-233). New York: Brunner/Mazel.

Blenkner, M. (1965). Social work and family relationships in later life with some thoughts on filial maturity. In E. Shanas & G. F. Streib (Eds.), *Social structure and the family: Generational relations.* Englewood Cliffs, NJ: Prentice-Hall.

Breslau, L. (1987). Exaggerated helplessness syndrome in the elderly. In J. Sadavoy & M. Leszcz (Eds.), *Treating the elderly with psychotherapy: The scope for change in later life* (pp. 157-173). Madison, CT: International Universities Press.

Burnside, I. (1984). *Working with the elderly: Group process and techniques* (2nd ed.). Monterey, CA: Wadsworth Health Sciences Division.

Butler, R. N., & Lewis, M. I. (1973). *Aging and mental health: Positive psychosocial approaches.* St. Louis: Mosby.

Cath, S. H. (1965). Some dynamics of middle and later years: A study in depletion and restitution. In M. A. Berezin & S. H. Cath (Eds.), *Geriatric psychiatry: Grief, loss and emotional disorders in the aging process* (pp. 21-72). New York: International Universities Press.

Cath, S. H. (1976). Functional disorders: An organismic view and attempt at reclassification. In L. Bellak & T. B. Karasu (Eds.), *Geriatric psychiatry—A handbook for psychiatrists and primary care physicians* (pp. 141-172). New York: Grune & Stratton.

Cohen, N. A. (1982). On loneliness and the aging process. *Int J Psychoanal, 63*, 149.

Erikson, E. H. (1968). The human life cycle. In D. L. Sills (Ed.), *International Encyclopedia of the Social Sciences* (pp. 286-292). New York: Macmillan.

Gaitz, C. M. (1974). Barriers to the delivery of psychiatric services to the elderly. *Gerontologist, 14,* 210-214.

Gallagher, D., & Thompson, L. W. (1982a). Cognitive therapy for depression in the elderly: A promising model for treatment and research. In L. Breslau & M. Haug (Eds.), *Depression and aging: Causes, care, and consequences* (pp. 168-192). New York: Springer.

Gallagher, D., & Thompson, L. W. (1982b). Differential effectiveness of psychotherapies for the treatment of major depressive disorders in older adult patients. *Psychotherapy: Theory, Research and Practice, 19,* 482-490.

Goldfarb, A. I. (1956). Psychotherapy of the aged: The use and value of an adaptational frame of reference. *Psychoanal Rev, 43,* 168-181.

Gotestam, K. G. (1980). Behavioral and dynamic psychotherapy with the elderly. In J. E. Birren & R. B. Sloan (Eds.), *Mental health and aging* (pp. 775-805). Englewood Cliffs, NJ: Prentice-Hall.

Grunes, J. (1987). The aged in psychotherapy: Psychodynamic contributions to the treatment process. In J. Sadavoy & M. Leszcz (Eds.), *Treating the elderly with psychotherapy: The scope for change in later life* (pp. 31–44). Madison, CT: International Universities Press.

Hartford, M. E. (1980). The use of group methods for work with the aged. In J. E. Birren & R. B. Sloan (Eds.), *Mental health and aging* (pp. 806–862). Englewood Cliffs, NJ: Prentice-Hall.

Hiatt, H. (1971). Dynamic psychotherapy with the aging patient. *Am J Psychother, 25,* 591–600.

Kahana, R. J. (1979). Strategies of dynamic psychotherapy with a wide range of older individuals. *J Geriatr Psychiat, 12*(1), 71–99.

Kahana, R. J. (1987). Geriatric psychotherapy: Beyond crisis management. In J. Sadavoy & M. Leszcz (Eds.), *Treating the elderly with psychotherapy: The scope for change in later life* (pp. 233–263). Madison, CT: International Universities Press.

Karasu, T. B. (1986). The specificity versus nonspecificity dilemma: Toward identifying therapeutic change agents. *Am J Psychiatry, 143*(6), 687–695.

Karasu, T. B., & Waltzman, S. A. (1976). Dying, death, and funerals. In L. Bellak & T. B. Karasu (Eds.), *Geriatric psychiatry—A handbook for psychiatrists and primary care physicians* (pp. 247–278). New York: Grune & Stratton.

King, P. H. M. (1974). Notes on the psychoanalysis of older patients. *J Analytical Psycholog, 19,* 22–37.

King, P. H. M. (1980). The life cycle as indicated by the nature of the transference in the psychoanalysis of the middle-aged and elderly. *Int J Psychoanal, 61,* 153–159.

Kohut, H. (1977). *Restoration of the self*. New York: International Universities Press.

Lawton, M. P. (1976). Geropsychological knowledge as a background for psychotherapy with older people. *J Geriatr Psychiat, 9,* 221–233.

Lazarus, L. W. (1980). Self psychology and psychotherapy with the elderly: Theory and practice. *J Geriatr Psychiat, 13,* 69–88.

Lazarus, L. W., & Groves, L. (1987). Brief psychotherapy with the elderly: A study of process and outcome. In J. Sadavoy & M. Leszcz (Eds.), *Treating the elderly with psychotherapy: The scope for change in later life* (pp. 265–293). Madison, CT: International Universities Press.

Lazarus, L. W., & Weinberg, J. (1980). Treatment in the ambulatory care setting. In E. W. Busse & D. Blazer (Eds.), *Handbook of geriatric psychiatry* (pp. 427–452). New York: Van Nostrand Reinhold.

Leszcz, M. (1987). Group psychotherapy with the elderly. In J. Sadavoy & M. Leszcz (Eds.), *Treating the elderly with psychotherapy: The scope for change in later life* (pp. 325–349). Madison, CT: International Universities Press.

Leszcz, M., Feigenbaum, E., Sadavoy, J., & Robinson, A. (1985). A men's group. Psychotherapy with elderly men. *Internat J Group Psychother, 35*(2), 177–196.

Lewis, M. I., & Butler, R. N. (1974). Life-review therapy: Putting memories to work in individual and group psychotherapy. *Geriatrics, 29,* 11.

McEwan, E. G. (1987). The whole grandfather: An intergenerational approach to family therapy. In J. Sadavoy & M. Leszcz (Eds.), *Treating the elderly with psychotherapy: The scope for change in later life* (pp. 295–324). Madison, CT: International Universities Press.

Meerloo, J. A. M. (1961). Modes of psychotherapy in the aged. *J Amer Geriatr Soc, 9*, 225–234.

Meissner, W. W. (1975, November). *Normal psychology of the aging process revisited—I. Discussion.* Paper presented at the annual scientific meeting of the Boston Society of Gerontologic Psychiatry.

Muslin, H., & Epstein, L. J. (1980). Preliminary remarks on the rationale for psychotherapy of the aged. *Comp Psychiat, 21*(1), 1–12.

Myers, W. A. (1984). *Dynamic therapy for the older patient.* New York: Aronson.

Nagy, I., & Spark, G. M. (1973). *Invisible loyalties: Reciprocity in intergenerational family therapy.* Hagerstown, MD: Harper & Row.

Nemiroff, R. A., & Colarusso, C. A. (1985). *The race against time: Psychotherapy and psychoanalysis in the second half of life.* New York: Plenum.

Pfeiffer, E. (1971). Psychotherapy with elderly patients. *Postgraduate Medicine, 50*, 254–258.

Pollock, G. H. (1982). On aging and psychopathology. *Int J Psychoanal, 63*, 275–281.

Pollock, G. H. (1987). The mourning-liberation process: Ideas on the inner life of the older adult. In J. Sadavoy & M. Leszcz (Eds.), *Treating the elderly with psychotherapy: The scope for change in later life* (pp. 3–29). Madison, CT: International Universities Press.

Rechtschaffen, A. (1959). Psychotherapy with geriatric patients: A review of the literature. *J Gerontology, 14*, 73–84.

Ripeckyj, A. J., & Lazarus, L. W. (1984). Management of old age: Psychotherapy: Individual, group and family. In D. W. K. Kay & G. D. Burrows (Eds.), *Handbook of studies on psychiatry and old age* (pp. 375–386). Amsterdam, The Netherlands: Elsevier Science Publishers.

Sadavoy, J. (1987). Character disorders in the elderly: An overview. In J. Sadavoy & M. Leszcz (Eds.), *Treating the elderly with psychotherapy: The scope for change in later life* (pp. 175–229). Madison, CT: International Universities Press.

Sadavoy, J., & Dorian, B. (1983). Treatment of the elderly characterologically disturbed patient in the chronic care institution. *J Geriatr Psychiat, 16*(2), 223–240.

Shanas, E. (1984). Old parents and middle-aged children: The four and five generation family. *J Geriatr Psychiat, 17*(1), 7–19.

Steuer, J., Mintz, J., Hammen, C. L., Hill, M. A., Jarvik, L. F., McCarley, T., Motoike, P., & Rosen, R. (1984). Cognitive-behavioral and psychodynamic group psychotherapy in treatment of geriatric depression. *J Consult and Clinical Psychol, 52*, 180–189.

Sussman, M. B. (1965). Relationships of adult children with their parents in the United States. In E. Shanas & G. F. Streib (Eds.), *Social structure and the family: Generational relationships.* Englewood Cliffs, NJ: Prentice-Hall.

Thompson, L. W., Gallagher, D., & Breckenridge, J. S. (1987). Comparative effectiveness of psychotherapies for depressed elders. *J Consult and Clinical Psychol, 55*(3), 385-390.

Yesavage, J. A., & Karasu, T. B. (1982). Psychotherapy with elderly patients. *Am J Psychother, 36*(1), 41-55.

9
Somatic Therapies in Geriatric Psychiatry

Charles A. Shamoian

Psychiatric problems of the elderly, as with any age group, are amenable to treatment by the usual therapeutic modalities, including the somatic therapies. However, because of the aging process and superimposed multiple medical illnesses, specific knowledge in the application of these therapies to the elderly is required. This chapter will review the major principles for the use of the classes of psychopharmacological agents and electroconvulsive therapy in elderly patients.

I. General Principles Regarding Psychopharmacologic and Electroconvulsive Therapy (Blumenthal, 1982; Crook, Ferris, & Bartus, 1983; Jenike, 1985; Salzman, 1984)

A. Organic therapies are often used indiscriminately or unnecessarily in the elderly (especially medications). When used knowledgeably and appropriately they can reduce suffering and save lives.
B. Before instituting organic therapies the following should be considered:
   1. Many medical and neurological illnesses may present as psychiatric signs and symptoms and vice versa. Therefore, an adequate, comprehensive recent evaluation of medical and, when indicated, neurological studies should be performed.
   2. For patients presenting with chronic mental disorders, especially dementia, thorough medical, neurological, and psychiatric eval-

uations are critical to rule out causes for which specific treatments exist (e.g., apathetic hyperthyroidism, meningioma, major depressive episode, drug effect, etc.).
3. Rating scales are available that can serve as objective measures and document the severity of impairment and progression [e.g., Hamilton, Beck, Sandoz Clinical Assessment-Geriatric Scale (SCAGS), Mini-Mental State Exam (MMS), Kahn-Goldfarb, Global Assessment Scale, Brief Psychiatric Rating Scale (BPRS), etc.].
4. What are the risk/benefit ratios in view of possible side effects, interactions with other treatments, likelihood that treatment will be effective, relapse rates, and the support system available to the patient?

II. Psychopharmacologic Treatment

A. General Considerations (Jarvik & Small, 1982; Jenike, 1985; Salzman, 1984; Vestal, 1978)
1. Is the psychiatric disturbance caused or aggravated by medications prescribed by one or more physicians, or by medications obtained over-the-counter or from friends? The elderly frequently experience more side effects from CNS drugs than younger individuals.
2. Compliance problems are common with all patients and include taking too few or too many medications, particularly in the presence of early dementia, multiple medications, frequent administration, and unpleasant side effects. The elderly often use outdated drugs, share medications, purchase inappropriate over-the-counter (OTC) preparations, and obtain prescriptions from several physicians.
3. Polypharmacy is a serious problem, not only because of the multiple illnesses and multiple physicians involved in many cases, but also because of the vulnerability to side effects, including confusion, iatrogenic illness, and drug–drug interactions that interfere with therapeutic effects.
4. The physician should bear in mind the desirability of obtaining a complete drug history, discontinuing medications whenever possible, and minimizing concomitant use of several drugs.
5. When prescribing medications, the physician should be aware of the value of specific details concerning the type and purpose of the medications, the exact techniques (such as with meals, before bedtime, not with antacid, etc.), strategies for counting and

monitoring pills for patients with cognitive difficulties, and limiting prescriptions to small quantities to reduce the risk of lethal overdoses.
   6. Frequent visits to the psychiatrist to monitor side effects, listening to the patient and significant others, and reassurance regarding the psychiatrist's availability are important. All these considerations facilitate the care of the geriatric patient.
B. Pharmacokinetics (Crooks, 1976; Greenblatt & Koch-Weser, 1975) is the study and characterization of the time course of drug absorption, distribution, metabolism, and excretion and is concerned with the relationship of these processes to the intensity and time course of therapeutics and adverse effects of drug. Aging affects many of these variables, including the drug availability to the brain. Knowledge of pharmacokinetics tends to enhance effective treatment and to minimize side effects. Pharmacodynamics is defined as the study of drug action at the receptor and the subsequent effects of that action.
   1. Age-related changes in absorption may be very significant for vitamins and minerals because they require active transport, but relatively insignificant for psychotropic medications, which are absorbed largely by diffusion. These age-related changes that affect absorption include:
      a. Increase in gastric ph.
      b. Decrease in intestinal blood flow.
      c. Decreases in absorption caused by the use of antacids, by congestive heart failure, and by anticholinergic slowing of gastric motility.
      d. By contrast, an empty stomach generally tends to enhance absorption.
   2. Drug distribution is often altered because of aging. Significant changes include:
      a. Total body water decreases, causing increased plasma levels and toxicity of water soluble drugs (e.g., lithium).
      b. Lean body mass decreases with associated increase in percentage of body fat, leading to longer half-life, and prolonged clearance, of lipid soluble drugs (antipsychotics, antidepressants, and antianxiety drugs).
      c. Plasma albumin levels decrease and may result in increased concentrations of free active drug for many psychoactive drugs (e.g., amitriptyline, nortriptyline, imipramine, desipramine, doxepin, Dilantin, etc.)
   3. Metabolism of drugs decreases because of reduced hepatic enzy-

matic activity and diminished hepatic blood flow. The first-pass effect is reduced, especially in the presence of such pathological states as congestive heart failure and hepatic disease.
4. Remember that only water soluble medications, such as lithium, are detoxified by renal excretion. Other psychotropic medications are detoxified in the liver and then excreted by the kidney.
    a. According to cross-sectional studies, renal function (both glomerular filtration rate and renal plasma flow) normally diminishes by approximately 1% each year after age 30. Renal function is further impaired by dehydration, hypotension, and congestive heart failure. Since blood creatinine may be decreased because of reduced muscle mass, it is not a reliable measure of renal function, and creatinine clearance may have to be determined.
    b. For lithium, there is lower clearance and longer time required to achieve steady state in the elderly compared to young adults.
5. Neuron receptor changes include increased sensitivity to benzodiazepines and lithium, with toxicity occurring at lower plasma drug levels compared to young adults.
6. Pathological states such as malnutrition can lower albumin levels, increasing further the levels of unbound, active, free drug.
7. In general, all of these pharmacokinetic changes may delay onset of drug effects, prolong the effect (for some medications, such as long-acting benzodiazepines, half-life may be increased to several weeks), increase the plasma level, enhance or interfere with the response, and result in toxicity.

C. Antipsychotic Medications—Neuroleptics
1. The various classes of antipsychotics (phenothiazines, butyrophenones, thiothixenes) tend to be similar in efficacy, but differ in side effects and potency per mgm. The choice of medication usually depends on the side-effect profile (e.g, the side effect the treating psychiatrist wishes to avoid in a particular patient).
2. The primary indications for use of the drugs include acute psychiatric episodes and maintenance for chronic state of schizophrenia; delusional (paranoid) disorders; acute stage of bipolar disorders—manic; major depressive episode, mood-congruent psychotic features, delirium, and psychoses of dementia.
3. Demented patients without agitation and psychosis, patients with acute alcohol withdrawal states, with decompensated untreated cardiac conditions (such as complete heart block, sick sinus syndrome), with Parkinsonism, and patients taking sedatives, alcohol, and analgesics can usually be managed without neuroleptics.

4. Whenever possible, use lowest doses and if necessary increase gradually. Monitoring of blood pressure and side effects is recommended; rapidly changing from one drug to another is to be avoided, if possible, since this can result in inadequate treatment; collaborate with support network (e.g., family, nurses) to observe side effects and increase compliance.
5. Plasma levels vary markedly between individuals, for different medications, and do not necessarily correlate with therapeutic response; they may be useful when overdose or failure to take medications is suspected.
6. Although there are many possible side effects, the common ones are extrapyramidal, anticholinergic, and cardiovascular. Others include lowered seizure threshold, agranulocytosis, sexual dysfunction, photosensitivity, and neuroleptic malignant syndrome.
   a. These extrapyramidal symptoms (EPS) can be especially disabling in the presence of other musculoskeletal disorders (such as amyotrophic lateral sclerosis, rheumatoid arthritis, and Parkinson's disease).
      (1) The parkinsonian syndrome can include akinesia, bradykinesia, cogwheeling, drooling, falling, and difficulty in walking, drinking, and chewing.
      (2) Akathisia consists of motor restlessness, ranging from inner disquiet to inability to lie or sit still.
      (3) Dystonic reactions include muscular rigidity and can include oculogyric crises and opisthotonos.
      (4) Tardive dyskinesia (TD) (Bernstein, 1982) includes athetoid-choreic movements, most frequently of the mouth and tongue (buccal-lingual) but also of the trunk and limbs. It can occur after long-term use of antipsychotic drugs but can also appear after a short period with high-potency antipsychotics. Ill-fitting dentures can induce similar muscular movements. Five percent of the elderly never exposed to neuroleptics spontaneously develop TD movements.
         (a) No definitive treatment for TD is currently available.
         (b) Approximately two-thirds of TD cases in the elderly appear to be irreversible (Smith & Baldessarini, 1980).
         (c) Recommended treatment includes gradually discontinuing anticholinergic drugs, followed by gradual lowering and discontinuation of antipsychotic medications, if possible. The TD symptoms may get worse initially, but then may disappear.
         (d) Discussing with patients and caregivers the advan-

tages and disadvantages of continuing and discontinuing medications is often helpful in the decision-making process.
  b. Anticholinergic symptoms include blurred vision, aggravation of narrow-angle glaucoma; dry mouth, tachycardia; constipation, which may lead to bowel obstruction and ileus, urinary retention, and "atropinic" psychosis or toxic confusional state.
     (1) An "atropinic" psychosis can occur with antipsychotic, antidepressant, or anticholinergic medications, especially with combinations of drugs with CNS anticholinergic effects. It is characterized by the above symptoms plus delirium, anhidrosis, and hyperthermia. Recommended treatment consists of discontinuing medications and, in emergency, instituting proper life supports, including I.V. physostigmine with cardiac monitoring because of potential cardiac side effects of physostigmine.
  c. Cardiovascular problems (Hollister, 1978), including cardiac arrhythmias and orthostatic hypotension, can occur with any antipsychotic medication, but it is generally believed that high-potency drugs are safer than low-potency neuroleptics. Sudden death has rarely been reported with high-potency medications.
     (1) All neuroleptics can produce an alpha-adrenergic blockade with central and peripheral hypotension and reflex tachycardia.
     (2) Quinidine-like effects have been reported. These may resemble the effects of myocardial ischemia and lead to erroneous diagnosis of myocardial infarction.
  d. Neuroleptic malignant syndrome (Caroff, 1980) is characterized by muscular rigidity, akinesia, often with catatonic posturing, hyperthermia (101–106 degrees), and altered consciousness with the potential for stupor and coma. Labile blood pressure, diaphoresis, sialorrhea, incontinence, dysphasia, and dyskinesia are also noted. The syndrome occurs especially in males and younger patients. Oldest patient reported was 61, although cases in patients as old as 80 have been observed. Mortality rates of 20–30% have been associated with the syndrome.
     (1) Treatment includes discontinuing antipsychotic medications, maintaining hydration and electrolyte balance, reducing fever. Pneumonia and pulmonary emboli have been reported as complications.

(2) Although drugs such as bromocriptine and dantrolene have been used, as well as ECT, no definitive treatment is currently available.
7. Maintenance therapy must be carefully considered, and the decision is clinically determined since no long-term studies with elderly patients are available. The factors to be evaluated in making this decision include the past history (i.e., frequency and intensity of psychotic episodes) and effectiveness of the medication in preventing relapses. Periodic gradual tapering off of medication when clinically appropriate is suggested.
8. In some states (e.g., Massachusetts) it is necessary to have "substitute judgment" (permission from a judge) as well as permission from the next of kin or legal guardian to treat with antipsychotic medications except in emergencies when probable eminent harm may occur if patient is not treated with a neuroleptic.

D. Antidepressant medications (Bernstein, 1982; Cole, 1983; Gerner, 1983; Jarvik & Kakkar, 1981, Jenike, 1985; Salzman, 1984) include the polycyclic antidepressants, monoamine oxidase inhibitors, lithium, and stimulants.
1. Polycyclic antidepressants include tertiary amines (amitriptyline, doxepin, imipramine, trimipramine), secondary amines (nortriptyline, protriptyline, desipramine), and the newer second-generation antidepressants (amoxapine, maprotiline, trazodone, fluoxetine, etc.).
   a. Treatment indications include major depressive episode, with psychotic feature and/or with melancholia; bipolar disorder, depressed; depressive disorder, single or recurrent episodes; organic affective disorder.
   b. Contraindications include severe cardiac disease (sick sinus syndrome, complete heart block), immediately post CVA and immediately post MI, history of severe adverse reactions (i.e., agranulocytosis) to a particular antidepressant, and intracranial tumor.
   c. The drugs tend to be similar in efficacy but differ in side effects, such as sedation, hypotension, and anticholinergic effects.
   d. The secondary amines, desipramine and nortriptyline, are frequently used in the elderly, as well as trazodone and maprotiline. The tertiary amines are not used that often, primarily because of their hypotensive effects.
   e. Which drug and what dosage of that drug to use will be determined in part by the patient's past history or history of family members (Friedel, 1981, 1982).

(1) Usually small divided doses are used to reduce side effects and the dosage is gradually increased.
(2) The general consensus is that one medication should not be discontinued rapidly for another.
(3) There is marked variability to clinical response.
(4) Plasma levels need not be used routinely but may be useful in nonresponders to determine compliance or in suspected overdosage.
(5) Refractory patients may require a trial of several different medications, but each one should be used at appropriate dosages and for sufficient periods (e.g., sometimes up to two to three weeks) before considering the drug trial a failure.
  f. Side effects (Bernstein, 1982; Cassem, 1982; Glassman et al., 1982; Preskorn & Iruris, 1983)
    (1) Cardiovascular side effects include postural hypotension, dizziness, sinus tachycardia, and quinidine-like effects. The tricyclic antidepressants appear to have antiarrhythmic properties but can, in the overdose situation, cause atrial or ventricular premature contractions. *Caution*: Medical clearance before administering is recommended for patients with severe cardiac disease.
    (2) Anticholinergic side effects are described above in antipsychotic section 6b.
    (3) Neurological side effects include tremor, twitches, jitteriness, paresthesias, weakness, and ataxia.
    (4) Gastrointestinal side effects include constipation, ileus, nausea, vomiting, heartburn, and weight gain.
  g. Maintenance treatment is determined primarily by the patient's past history of affective episodes and response to treatment. In the elderly, studies are not conclusive and maintenance dosage is determined empirically. Doses as low as 25 mg per day of tricyclics may be effective. The rule of thumb, derived from studies on younger patients, is that patients should remain on maintenance dosages for six months to one year before the antidepressant is gradually tapered and then discontinued.
2. Monoamine oxidase inhibitors (MAOI) (Ashford & Ford, 1979; Bernstein, 1983; Jenike, 1985; Lazarus et al., 1986; Robinson, 1981, 1982; Salzman, 1984) include hydrazine (phenelzine, isocarboxazid) and nonhydrazine MAOIs (tranylcypromine, pargyline). Because MAO activity in the brain increases with aging, these drugs may be particularly effective in the elderly. How-

ever, because of hypertensive crises due to ingestion of tyramine-containing foods or over-the-counter preparations containing epinephrine–norepinephrine derivatives, these medications are usually reserved for patients who are highly motivated and have a strong support system.
  a. Indications include atypical depression, which is characterized by anxiety, obsessions, phobias, agoraphobia, hypochondriasis, fatigue, anergia, and hypersomnolence. Also, as a second choice after a patient has failed to respond to tricyclics and to second-generation antidepressants.
  b. Contraindications include severe liver disease, concomitant use of narcotic analgesics such as meperidine, patients who are not compliant with tyramine-free diet, and patients who require sympathomimetic medications.
  c. The physician should carefully outline the dietary regimen and types of medications to be avoided. Also, the signs and symptoms of hypertension (blurred vision, throbbing occipital headache) are to be explained as well as what to do in an emergency; that is, discontinuing medications and immediately going to an emergency room. Patients ingesting MAOIs often carry a card stating the specific MAOI they are ingesting and the drugs to be avoided in case of an emergency.
  d. Sudden orthostatic hypotension probably occurs more often than hypertensive crises and can be life-threatening in the elderly.
  e. Dosage of MAOIs varies according to the specific drug (i.e., usual daily dosage for phenelzine is 30–60 mg per day and for pargyline it is 10–25 mg per day). As with all medications in the elderly, the patient is started on small divided doses and increased gradually to the recommended limit or therapeutic response. If given in the morning and afternoon, insomnia can often be avoided.
  f. Major side effects include, in addition to the hypertensive reaction and orthostatic hypotension, hypomania, weight gain, impotence, gastrointestinal disturbance, drowsiness, and sleep disturbance.
  g. Use of polycyclics and MAOIs simultaneously is generally not recommended. However, this combination has been used in very resistant cases. The combination of these drugs may result in an increased incidence and severity of side effects. Studies using this combination in the elderly are lacking.
3. Stimulants (Kaufman, Cassem, Murray, & Jenike, 1984; Lehman & Ban, 1975; Salzman, 1979, 1981), including amphetamine,

methylphenidate, and pemoline, have been used to treat depression, but properly controlled clinical studies in the elderly are lacking.
   a. Indications (Kaufman et al., 1984) reported are: medically ill patients with a depression masked by the medical illness; depression following a stroke; the facilitation of rehabilitation of elderly patients with chronic illness; dementia and coexistent depression; and when ECT is contraindicated or when permission for its use is not forthcoming.
   b. Dosage usually recommended for methylphenidate is 20 to 40 mg per day. The beginning dose is usually 10 to 15 mg per day, with increments every day or two of 5 mg. The medication is usually given just before meals; if there is no therapeutic response within 48 to 72 hours, it is usually discontinued. The duration of treatment is empirical and individualized.
   c. Side effects include decreased appetite, insomnia, anxiety, agitation, loss of behavioral control, cardiac stimulation, myocardial infarction and cardiovascular accident, toxic psychosis, addiction, and rebound depression after discontinuation. These are usually noted after prolonged use. Data for elderly patients is lacking.
E. Lithium (Dunner, 1982; Foster, Gershell, & Goldfarb, 1977; Himmelhock, Neil, May, Fuchs, & Licata, 1980; Jenike, 1985; Prien, 1981)
   1. The indications for lithium use are bipolar disorder, particularly maintenance and prophylaxis; for acute manic episodes which may also require use of neuroleptics to quickly control symptoms; for recurrent major depressive episodes. Its effectiveness as an antidepressant during the early stages of an acute onset of depression is equivocal. Other indications include polycyclic-resistant depressions.
   2. Relative contraindications include patients with renal disease, on salt-free diets and diuretics. In these states, lithium clearance is reduced and toxicity can quickly ensue. Also, untreated hypothyroidism and cardiovascular disorder such as the sick sinus syndrome are relative contraindications.
   3. Prelithium evaluation includes CBC, BUN, electrolytes, creatinine clearance, thyroid function tests, urinalysis, and EKG. Without focal neurologic signs, an EEG is usually not required.
   4. Dosage must be carefully titrated in the elderly, since the half-life is prolonged.
      a. The dosage is started low, 75 to 300 mg per day, and increased by approximately 75 mg to 150 mg every two to

three days. The latter is based on an elimination half-life in the elderly of approximately 36 hours.
   b. A therapeutic response may take longer than the usual time in younger patients.
   c. Plasma levels less than 0.7 mEg/l may achieve therapeutic response and maintenance. However, the plasma levels required for maintenance should be individualized. Some elderly patients may require plasma levels as low as 0.30 mEg/l.
5. Monitoring lithium levels and clinical evaluations generally are performed more frequently in the elderly as compared to younger patients.
   a. Initially, during the acute illness, serum levels may need to be obtained every few days and then weekly or biweekly.
   b. After stabilization, levels are usually obtained monthly.
   c. If renal function is normal, serum creatine and BUN are usually monitored on a semiannual basis.
6. Side Effects
   a. At therapeutic plasma levels, side effects include polydipsia, polyuria, nausea, diarrhea, tremors, dizziness, weight gain, edema, hypothyroidism, goiter, skin rash, loss of hair, and fluid retention. Occasionally there is a decreased ability to concentrate urine (nephrogenic diabetes insipidus), which may be responsive to dosage adjustment or thiazides. The question of possible renal damage from lithium has not been clarified. Cardiac effects include EKG changes such as ST-T wave changes and conduction disturbances.
   b. At toxic levels nausea, vomiting, diarrhea, coarse tremors, sleeepiness, vertigo, and dysarthria are noted and progress to cardiac arrhythmias, confusion, disorientation, delirium, muscle fasciculation, hyperreflexia, convulsions, oliguria, anuria, and death.
   c. Maintenance therapy decreases frequency and severity of episodes of mania and depression. Duration of maintenance therapy in the elderly is determined by frequency of prior episodes and response to lithium. The possibility of renal pathology during lithium maintenance may be determined by yearly creatinine clearance. Also, thyroid function may be periodically evaluated by measuring serum thyroxine (T_4), L-triodothyronine (T_3), and thyroid stimulating hormone (TSH).
F. Antianxiety agents (Bernstein, 1983) include benzodiazepines, barbiturates, glycerol derivatives (meprobamate), and antihistamines.
   1. Indications include acute and chronic anxiety, anxiety-depression syndrome, alcohol withdrawal, and acute agitation.

2. Relative contraindications include suicidal or severely depressed patients, CNS depression, including that induced by alcohol, and serious pulmonary disorders.
3. Dosage should begin with small doses and be gradually increased until therapeutic response is achieved. Short-acting benzodiazepines (alprazolam, temazepam, and oxazepam) are preferable to long-acting medications (diazepam, chlordiazepoxide) for daily usage. Multiple daily dosages of long-acting benzodiazepines can result in accumulation of the drug and cause ataxia, falls, sedation, depression, and confusion.
4. Side effects include sedation, ataxia, confusion, aggressive behavior, and tolerance to the medication.
5. Maintenance with barbiturates, benzodiazepines, and glycerol derivatives should be avoided if possible. If absolutely necessary, medication should be gradually decreased to determine the need for continuing maintenance. Long-term usage can lead to tolerance and addiction. Abrupt withdrawal may lead to seizures and symptoms similar to those for which the antianxiety agent was originally prescribed.

G. Sedative-hypnotics (Feinberg & Koegler, 1982; Shader, 1982) most commonly used are benzodiazepines, halogenated hydrocarbon (chloral hydrate), and antihistamines (diphenhydramine), but many others exist, including barbiturates, piperidinediones (glutethimide), quinazolones (methaqualone), and higher alcohols (ethchlorvynol).
1. If possible, initially medications should be avoided and nonpharmacologic approaches instituted, including:
    a. Educating the elderly patient; that is, they sleep lighter, sleep less, and awaken more often than younger people.
    b. Avoiding daytime napping.
    c. Exercising regularly during the day.
    d. Avoiding caffeine, nicotine, and alcohol and restricting fluid intake.
    e. Controlling nighttime pain.
2. The most commonly used sedative-hypnotics are flurazepam, oxazepam, temazepam, and triazolam. The shorter-acting temazepam and triazolam are preferable. Flurazepam has active metabolites and thus a very long-half life (up to weeks in the elderly).
3. Indications include early, middle, and late insomnia. Sleep disturbances due to depression, mania, paraphrenia, and psychosis are not treated per se but dissipate when the underlying psychiatric illness is appropriately treated with the indicated psychotropic.

4. *Caution*: Sedative-hypnotics, and specifically the benzodiazepines, are the most frequently prescribed and abused medications. With long-term use they are addicting and lose their effectiveness. As soon as possible, taper and discontinue benzodiazepines.
H. Memory-enhancement drugs (Neshkes & Jarvik, 1983; Reisberg, Ferris, & Gershon, 1981; Reisberg, London, Ferris, Anand, & deLeon, 1983; Branconnier, 1983; Johns, Greenwald, Mohs, & Davis, 1983) are used in the hope of reversing or stabilizing cognitive and memory loss usually found in the dementias. None has shown demonstrable efficacy. Yet some patients improve on these drugs, most of which remain experimental.
  1. Memory-enhancement drugs include vasodilators (niacin), cerebral stimulants (pentelenetetrazol), hormones (vasopressin and ACTH peptides), metabolic precursors (choline, lecithin, physostigmine), and metabolic enhancers (dihydroergotoxine mesylate).
  2. Dihydroergotoxine mesylate is the only FDA-approved drug currently available that may have some usefulness for some demented patients.

III. Electroconvulsive Therapy—ECT
(Bidder, 1981; Fink, 1982; Salzman, 1982a)

A. Indications
  1. Effective, reliable, and safe modality for treatment of acute mania and depression.
  2. Is used especially when antidepressant medications have failed, have caused complications, or are contraindicated because of medical illness.
  3. It has been recommended particularly for patients who are suicidal, cachectic, dehydrated, and delusional (especially delusions of guilt or somatic symptoms).
  4. Patients with neurovegetative signs and symptoms of depression often respond better than patients with a great degree of associated anxiety.
B. Prior to ECT, a medical evaluation—with baseline studies such as EKG, EEG, chest or lumbarsacral-spine x-ray, CBC, urinalysis, and appropriate blood chemistries—is appropriate and recommended.
C. An absolute contraindication is increased intracranial pressure. Relative contraindications include recent myocardial infarction, recent cerebrovascular accident, and severe hypertension because of an increased associated morbidity and mortality (APA Task Force on ECT, 1978).

D. Although the APA Task Force on ECT acknowledged that each individual psychiatrist should decide whether to use unilateral or bilateral ECT, it recommended use of unilateral ECT because of the lower potential for memory difficulty.
   1. Number of treatments is variable, usually between 6 and 20.
   2. The recommended treatment schedule is two to three per week.
   3. Reality orientation and milieu therapy in conjunction with ECT are recommended.
E. Complications may include fracture, seizure, amnesia, psychosis, and cardiac arrhthymia.
   1. These are infrequent, especially when patients are given a muscle relaxant and are adequately oxygenated.
   2. Mortality is less than 1 per 10,000 cases, which is lower than that associated with antidepressants.
   3. Cardiac monitoring during and immediately post-ECT is recommended for patients with cardiac problems.
F. Maintenance treatment (e.g., once per month on outpatient basis) is appropriate for patients who have responded to ECT and have relapses despite ongoing treatment with antidepressant medications.
G. Antidepressant nonresponders are usually considered for a course of ECT. Whether or not maintenance antidepressant treatments are effective in these patients after a course of ECT is not clear, especially for the elderly.

REFERENCES

American Psychiatric Task Force on ECT. (1978). *Electroconvulsive therapy*. Washington, DC: American Psychiatric Association.

Ashford, J. W., & Ford, C. V. (1979). Use of MAO inhibitors in elderly patients. *Am J Psychiatry, 136*, 1466–1467.

Bernstein, J. G. (1982). *Handbook of drug therapy in psychiatry*. Littleton, MA: John Wright.

Bernstein, J. G. (1983). *Handbook of drug therapy in psychiatry*. Littleton, MA: John Wright.

Bidder, T. G. (1981). Electroconvulsive therapy in the medically ill patient. In J. T. Strain (Ed.), *The psychiatric clinics of North America—The medically ill patient* (Volume 4:2). Philadelphia: Saunders.

Blumenthal, M. D. (1982). Drug treatment in elderly psychiatric patients. In C. Eisdorfer & W. E. Fann (Eds), *Treatment of psychopathology in the aging* (pp. 159–173). New York: Springer.

Branconnier, R. J. (1983). The efficacy of the cerebral metabolic enhancers in the treatment of senile dementia. *Psychopharmacology Bull, 19*, 212–219.

Caroff, S. N. (1980). The neuroleptic syndrome. *J Clin Psychiatry*, 41, 79–83.
Cassem, N. (1982). Cardiovascular effects of antidepressants. *J Clin Psychiatry*, 43, 22–28.
Cole, J. O. (1983). New antidepressant drugs. *McLean Hosp J*, 8, 62–77.
Crook, T., Ferris, S., & Bartus, R. (1983). *Assessment in geriatric psychopharmacology*. New Canaan, CT: Mark Powley.
Crooks, J., O'Malley, K. O., & Stevenson, I. H. (1976). Pharmacokinetics in the elderly. *Clinical Pharmacokinetics*, 1, 280–296.
Dunner, D. L. (1982). Lithium treatment of the aged. In C. Eisdorfer & W. E. Fann (Eds), *Treatment of psychopathology in the aging* (pp. 137–145). New York: Springer.
Feinberg, I., & Koegler, A. (1982). Hypnotics and the elderly: Clinical and basic science issues. In C. Eisdorfer & W. E. Fann (Eds.), *Treatment of psychopathology in the aging* (pp. 75–76). New York: Springer.
Fink, M. (1982). ECT in the elderly. In C. Eisdorfer & W. E. Fann (Eds.), *Treatment of psychopathology in the aging* (pp. 97–111). New York: Springer.
Foster, J., Gershell, W., & Goldfarb, A. (1977). Lithium treatment in the elderly. *J Gerontology*, 32, 299–302.
Friedel, R. O. (1981). Effects of age in the pharmacology of tricyclic antidepressants. In A. Raskin, D. S. Robinson, & J. Levine (Eds.), *Age and the pharmacology of psychoactive drugs* (pp. 125–132). New York: Elsevier.
Friedel, R. O. (1982). The relationship of therapeutic response to antidepressant plasma levels: An update. *J Clin Psychiatry*, 43, 37–42.
Gerner, R. H. (1983). Systemic treatment approach to depression and treatment resistant depression. *Psychiatric Annals*, 13, 37–49.
Gibaldi, M., & Levy, G. (1976). Pharmacokinetics in clinical practice. I. Concepts. *Journal of the American Medical Association*, 235, 1864–1867.
Glassman, A., Walsh, B. T., Roose, S. P., Rosenfeld, R., Bruno, R. L., Bigger, J. T., & Giardina, E. G. (1982). Factors related to orthostatic hypotension associated with tricyclic antidepressants. *J Clin Psychiatry*, 43, 35–38.
Greenblatt, D. J., & Divoll, M. (1982). Benzodiazepines in the elderly. In C. Eisdorfer & W. E. Fann (Eds.), *Treatment of psychopathology in the aging* (pp. 29–42). New York: Springer.
Greenblatt, D. J., & Koch-Weser, J. (1975). Clinical pharmacokinetics. *NEJM*, 293, 702–705.
Himmelhoch, J. M., Neil, J. F., May, S. J., Fuchs, C. Z., & Licata, S. M. (1980). Age, dementia, dyskinesia, and lithium response. *Am J Psychiatry*, 137, 941–945.
Hollister, L. E. (1978). *Clinical pharmacology of psychotherapeutic drugs*. New York: Churchill Livingstone.
Jarvik, L. F., & Kakkar, P. R. (1981). Aging and response to antidepressants. In L. F. Jarvik, D. Greenblatt, & D. Harmon (Eds.), *Clinical pharmacology and the aged patient* (pp. 49–77). *Aging: Vol. 16*. New York: Raven.
Jarvik, L. F., & Small, G. W. (1982). *Psychiatric clinics of North America: Vol. 5. Aging*. Philadelphia: Saunders.

Jenike, M. (1985). *Handbook of geriatric psychopharmacology*. Littleton, MA: PSG Publishing.

Johns, C. A., Greenwald, B. S., Mohs, R. C., & Davis, K. L. (1983). The cholinergic treatment strategy in aging and senile dementia. *Psychopharmacology Bull, 19*, 185-197.

Kaufman, M. W., Cassem, N. H., Murray, G. B., & Jenike, M. (1984). Use of psychostimulants in medically ill patients with neurological disease and major depression. *Can J Psychiatry, 29*, 46-49. 1984.

Lazarus, L. W., Groves, L., Gierl, B., Pandey, G., Javaid, J. I., Lesser, J., Hays, I., & Davis, J. (1986). Efficacy of phenelzine in geriatric depression. *Biological Psychiatry, 21*, 699-701.

Neshkes, R. E., & Jarvik, L. F. (1983). Pharmacologic approach to the treatment of senile dementia. *Psychiatric Annals, 13*, 14-30.

Preskorn, S. H., & Iruris, H. A. (1982). Toxicity of tricyclic antidepressants—Kinetics, mechanism, intervention: A review. *J Clin Psychiatry, 43*, 151-156.

Prien, R. D. (1981). Age related changes in lithium pharmacokinetics. In A. Raskin, D. S. Robinson, & J. Levine (Eds.), *Age and the pharmacology of psychoactive drugs* (pp. 163-169). New York: Elsevier.

Reisberg, B., Ferris, S. H., & Gershon, S. (1981). An overview of pharmacologic treatment of cognitive decline in the aged. *Am J Psychiatry, 138*, 595-600.

Reisberg, B., London, E., Ferris, S. H., Anand, R., & de Leon, M. J. (1983). Novel pharmacologic approaches to the treatment of senile dementia of the Alzheimer's type (SDAT). *Psychopharmacology Bull, 19*, 220-225.

Robinson, D. S. (1981). Monoamine oxidase inhibitors in the elderly. In A. Raskin, D. S. Robinson, & J. Levine (Eds.), *Age and the pharmacology of psychoactive drugs* (pp. 151-162). New York: Elsevier.

Robinson, D. S. (1982). Monoamine oxidase inhibitors in the elderly. In C. Eisdorfer & W. E. Fann (Eds.), *Treatment of psychopathology in the aging*. New York: Springer.

Salzman, C. (1979). Update on geriatric psychopharmacology. *Geriatrics, 34*, 87-90.

Salzman, C. (1981). Stimulants in the elderly. In A. Raskin, D. S. Robinson & J. Levine (Eds.), *Age and the pharmacology of psychoactive drugs* (pp. 171-180). New York: Elsevier.

Salzman, C. (1982a). Electronconvulsive therapy in the elderly patient. In L. F. Jarvik (Ed.), *The psychiatric clinics of North America—Aging* (Volume 5, #1) (pp. 191-197). Philadelphia: Saunders.

Salzman, C. (1982b). Psychotropic drug side effects in the elderly. In C. Eisdorfer & W. E. Fann (Eds.), *Treatment of psychopathology in the aging* (pp. 146-158). New York: Springer.

Salzman, C. (1984). *Clinical geriatric psychopharmacology*. New York: McGraw-Hill.

Shader, R. I., & Greenblatt, D. J. (1982). Management of anxiety in the elderly: The balance between therapeutic and adverse effects. *J Clin Psychiatry, 43*, 8-16.

Smith, J. M., & Baldessarini, R. J. (1980). Changes in prevalence, severity, and recovery in tardive dyskinesia with age. *Arch Gen Psychiatry, 37*, 1368.

Vestal, R. E. (1978). Drug use in the elderly: A review of problems and special considerations. *Drugs, 16*, 358-382.

10

The Organization of Mental Health Services for the Elderly

Barry Gurland, John Toner, Anthony Mustille, George Alexopoulos, Barry Fogel, Gary Gottlieb, John Barsa, Carl Cohen, Peter Birkett, Barry Meyers, Abraham Monk, Lois Grau, and John Copeland

There does not yet exist in this country a comprehensive system of mental health care for the elderly. Yet the creation of such a system should be a main objective of the organization of services. To achieve this objective will require defining the components and mechanisms that can add up to a good system of care, examining examples of successful efforts to put in place and integrate the elements of a system, and identifying means of resolving difficulties in the way of improving, expanding, and generalizing these efforts. In this direction a symposium was held in October 1986 that stimulated discussion, amongst a multidisciplinary group concerned with the mental health of the elderly, on the desirability, feasibility, obstacles, progress, and achievements in building a complete system of mental health care for the elderly. The sections that follow are selected, brief abstracts from

This outline is abstracted from an invitational conference on Building a Complete System of Mental Health Care for the Elderly, held on October 15th, 1986, under the auspices of the Columbia University Center for Geriatrics, the InterUniversity Consortium of Academic GeroPsychiatry, the New York State Geriatric Psychiatric Fellowship Program (Willard Psychiatric Center and the New York State Psychiatric Institute), and the Geriatric Subcommittee for Long Range Planning at Columbia Presbyterian Medical Center. The author of each section is listed in parentheses after the main heading.

this symposium. Space limitations did not allow a full consideration of all important issues relevant to a system of care, but the sections when taken together allow a view of a comprehensive system of mental health care in the making.

An overview of the components and connecting elements of a model geriatric mental health system is presented first; *selected* components are described subsequently. The programs described may have applicability to other settings.

I. The System of Care (B. Gurland)
(German, Shapiro, & Skinner, 1985; Hargreaves, 1986)

A. The treatment of mental disorders in aging patients is best managed with access to a system of care because:
  1. These disorders are complex, often extended in duration, and have changing needs over time.
  2. Many patients, such as relapsing depressives, aging schizophrenics, paraphrenics, and patients with progressive dementias will continue to grow old under the care of a psychiatrist.
  3. At some stage in the treatment of the aging patient, there may develop a complicating physical illness, an inability in tasks of self-care or independence, or multiple social problems. These, alone or in combination, might require referral to a geriatric psychiatrist or a multidisciplinary team, involvement of social services, acute hospital admission, or eventual change in residence, such as to a nursing home.
B. If treatment is not linked to a well organized system it can become:
  1. Time consuming.
  2. Disruptive of the ongoing relationship with the psychiatrist.
  3. Expensive.
  4. Inappropriate.
  5. Duplicative.
  6. Inconsistent.
C. It benefits each psychiatrist who treats elderly patients to be linked to a system of care and to understand this system or even to help to create it.
D. A system, according to the Concise Oxford Dictionary, is a set of connected things or parts.
E. Component sites of a mental health care system for the elderly include:
  1. Hospital or Institution Based
     a. Generic or psychiatric: tertiary, general (inpatient, acute, out-

patient, emergency), chronic, long-term care facility (nursing home/skilled nursing facility/SNF for mental disorders).
2. Dispersed Care Locations
   a. Medical (primary care, internists, other).
   b. Social (social services).
   c. Psychiatric (freestanding public, private psychiatrists).
3. Centralized Community Setting
   a. Medical (day hospital, health clinic).
   b. Social (senior center, daycare center, daycare for the confused).
   c. Psychiatric (day hospital, community mental health center, daycare for the confused with behavior problems, aftercare psychiatric clinic).
4. Congregate Residential Settings
   a. Senior housing, sheltered or enriched housing, halfway residences, homes for the aged.
   b. Shelters for the homeless, single-room-occupancy buildings.
   c. Shared housing, foster homes for the aged.
   d. Retirement communities, continuing care retirement communities.
   e. Prison.
5. Private Homes.
6. Streets and Public Places.

F. Component Linking, Coordinating, and Controlling Mechanisms
1. Aims:
   a. Linking services.
   b. Organizing transitions between services.
   c. Controlling allocation of resources.
   d. Monitoring operations.
   e. Guiding individuals through the system.
2. Methods:
   a. Interdisciplinary teams, joint medical and psychiatric units, liaison psychiatry, discharge planning, follow-up.
   b. Psychiatric outreach, medical and social consultation, mobile geriatric crisis units, home visiting, family services.
   c. Administrative management, case management, primary care, channeling/triage.
   d. Ombudsman/advocates, quality assurance, regulation, reimbursement rules.
   e. Resource allocation, manpower/training.
   f. Record linkages, information and referral.

II. Linkages and Coordination in Chronic Care Settings (A. Mustille)

A. A large, publicly supported psychiatric center can effectively direct a working system of mental health care for the elderly. The organizational perspective described here is based on the experience of a large psychiatric center in a rural location.
B. Scope of the problem: a center with a high concentration of elderly psychiatric patients may have a range of problems to deal with.
   1. Age of Patients
      a. Around two-thirds of the patients are over 65 years of age.
      b. The average age for females is 81 and for males, 74.
   2. Patients' Lack of Support Systems
      a. Ninety-five percent of patients are without a significant other who actively advocates for them.
      b. More than two-thirds are from outside the immediate catchment area.
   3. Patients' Physical Health
      a. About two-thirds of patients in the above-described setting are incontinent of urine.
      b. Half have limited ambulatory ability.
      c. A quarter require extra oral feedings.
      d. About a third are at risk for pressure ulcers.
      e. Ninety percent have one or more chronic physical illnesses in addition to their psychiatric disability.
   4. Patients' Mental Health
      a. Over one-half have long-term psychiatric disability.
      b. Severe dementia. More than a third of patients with a diagnosis of schizophrenia in remission carry a dual diagnosis of dementia.
C. Solutions to the above problems: to serve better these severely impaired elderly patients, the psychiatric center has organized a program composed of two major divisions:
   1. Pre- and posthospitalization (outpatient) programs.
   2. Hospitalization (inpatient) programs.
D. Criteria for Most Effective Programs
   1. Those that address a wide range of patient needs and serve the needs of the whole patient.
   2. Those programs that keep the patient in the natural environment the longest.
   3. Those programs that minimize as much as possible changes in the person's environment.
E. Examples of Programs

1. Admission/screening/referral services, which:
    a. Provide ongoing follow-up for caregivers.
    b. Link community care providers with the patient.
    c. Prevent inappropriate admissions: only about 1 in 12 patients who are screened need admission to the psychiatric center.
2. Certified clinic and continuing treatment programs offer:
    a. Assessment and treatment planning.
    b. Case management.
    c. Crisis services.
    d. Medication therapy.
    e. Verbal therapies.
    f. Social training.
    g. Care provided by an interdisciplinary team:
        (1) Headed by a psychiatrist.
        (2) A community mental health nurse provides medication education and, together with the social workers, offers supportive counseling as needed.
3. Family care programs: some patients reside in the community within a private home. Family care offers the elderly the supervision they may need with activities of daily living, medications, and socialization.
4. Personal care program: in some states, the personal care program is a Medicaid-reimbursable way of providing extra physical care and personal services (ADL/IADL) in a community-based residential option.
5. Preplacement program, involving:
    a. Easing the transitional period from institutional living to community residence.
    b. Inpatients attending group activities at the community outpatient centers.
    c. Establishing rapport with community providers of care and with patients living in the community.
6. Hospital industry program: a vocational program in collaboration with local industry that provides an opportunity for patients to learn work habits for pay.

F. Range of Coordinated Services Provided
   1. Assessment and Diagnostic Services
       a. A multidisciplinary approach.
       b. Diagnosis the responsibility of the psychiatrist/physician.
   2. Physical health screening and immunization: provides a data base for medical decisions and for determining the safety of the use of psychotropics.
   3. Structured Environment:

a. Reality orientation is provided.
   b. Provides an attitude of acceptance of behaviors such as wandering and sleep problems.
   c. Permits reduced use of medications.
  4. Opportunities for socialization.
  5. Adaptive equipment: facilitates ambulation and any degree of independence.
  6. Medical/nursing monitoring: early detection of infectious processes a primary consideration.
  7. Acute Medical Care
   a. At an onsite medical-surgical service.
   b. At hospitals in the community.
  8. Clinic services: provided by specialty consultants.
  9. Emergency services: advanced life support provided on site.
  10. Family support.
  11. Education: inservice education for nursing homes in the community as requested.
  12. Cooperative arrangement for referral and transfer of nursing home patients to the psychiatric center and vice versa:
   a. If the patient stabilizes within the time frame dictated by funding sources, the patient is returned to the "home."
   b. If the patient does not stabilize in that period, the "home" selects from a prescreened group of individuals who are psychiatrically stable but require residential care and a cooperative exchange is completed.
G. It is important to keep a system such as this flexible, with the emphasis on continuity of care, even though this emphasis may render the system cumbersome to administer and require that agencies involved conduct their business in ways best suited to the overall needs of the patient rather than those of the agency.

III. Private Psychiatric Hospitals (G. Alexopoulos)
(Finkel, 1983; Targum & Docherty, 1985)

A. A considerable number of patients with psychiatric disorders are treated in private institutions that may be profit or nonprofit oriented.
  1. These are usually organized around a general hospital.
  2. Those that are freestanding psychiatric hospitals, rather than part of a general hospital, have greater difficulty in maintaining high quality of care.
  3. Nonprofit institutions affiliated with medical schools are often in the avant-garde of medical education and research.

4. Profit-oriented hospitals tend to be relatively small and focused on care delivery in certain communities.
B. During the last decade, however, some profit-oriented hospitals:
   1. Have created "chains" of similar institutions.
   2. Have been a financial success when publicly supported institutions and many nonprofit voluntary hospitals have been facing major fiscal problems.
   3. Have in some instances developed programs of research.
C. The services provided by these private institutions depend to a large extent on their ability to at least meet their expenses:
   1. The population served by private hospitals is determined by their medical insurance status.
   2. Inpatient services are well developed.
   3. Other services are often limited to meeting the needs of patients after discharge.
   4. Community-oriented psychiatric services, such as outpatient departments, day hospitals, and outreach services, require a large trained staff and are therefore nonprofitable.
   5. The small number of services further restricts the population who can be treated.
D. Despite these limitations, a large number of geriatric patients can benefit from treatment in private institutions.
   1. Patients requiring complex tertiary care are candidates for treatment in large voluntary hospitals with advanced subspecialty services.
   2. Some medical centers have neuropsychiatric units where high-quality diagnostic evaluation and short-term treatment are offered to geriatric patients.
   3. Smaller hospitals treat geriatric psychiatric patients in nonspecialized inpatient psychiatric units.
   4. The availability of general hospital services permits diagnosis and treatment of disorders at the interface of psychiatry and medicine.
E. The relatively underdeveloped community services of private institutions complicate the care of geriatric psychiatric patients.
   1. Older individuals are unaccustomed to seeking help for psychiatric disorders and are less likely to enter the care delivery system of a private institution with poor outreach services.
   2. Depression and organic mental disorders, the most frequent psychiatric conditions in old age, interfere with the patient's initiative and ability to plan.
   3. Home visits or nursing home consultations are offered only by some hospitals because Medicare usually does not reimburse these services adequately.

4. Psychiatric outpatient services provided by private practitioners are poorly reimbursed by Medicare.
F. For all practical purposes, geriatric patients need to be able to cover part of their own expenses if they wish to be cared for by private psychiatrists.
G. In conclusion:
  1. Private institutions offer high-quality services for the psychiatric geriatric inpatient.
  2. Outpatient services are less available through the private sector.
  3. Care provided by private practitioners is restricted to persons who can afford it financially, unless the psychiatrist is willing to provide outpatient therapy for limited reimbursement from Medicare and other insurance carriers.

IV. The Medical-Psychiatric Inpatient Unit (B. Fogel) (Fogel & Stoudemire, 1986; Stoudemire & Fogel, 1986)

A. Medical-psychiatric units are inpatient facilities that are located in general hospitals and are oriented toward caring for patients with combined medical and psychiatric problems.
B. The staff of a medical-psychiatric unit must receive suitable training.
  1. Psychiatrists must have substantial knowledge of medicine and particular skills in applying psychopharmacologic treatments to the medically ill.
  2. Nursing staff must be trained in both medical and psychiatric assessment and intervention and be able to use occasions of physical care as an opportunity for psychotherapeutic and psychoeducational contact.
C. Medical-psychiatric units are ideal settings for the treatment of severe major depression occurring in the context of chronic medical illness.
  1. If managed by the psychiatric service, these units usually are DRG-exempt and therefore can offer lengths of stay of several weeks.
  2. The medical skills of nurses and the ready availability of medical consulting services permit greater safety in the use of psychotropic drugs and ECT than do traditional psychiatric units.
  3. Psychiatric side effects of medical drugs and somatic symptoms of depression are addressed by staff especially familiar with these problems.
  4. Family therapy and individual psychotherapy can focus effectively on adaptation to chronic illness.
  5. Time in hospital needed for medical stabilization can be used

simultaneously for psychotherapy, occupational therapy, and other therapies.
D. Patients with mental-status changes of unclear etiology can also be helped by a medical-psychiatric admission. To reach their highest level of function, these patients may require:
  1. Delicate adjustment of their medical regimen.
  2. Withdrawing and/or substituting drugs.
  3. Close observation of both the medical and psychiatric consequences of changes in regimen.
E. Outcome of Medical-Psychiatric Intervention
  1. This is usually good when patients have affective disorders or drug toxicity contributing to their functional decline.
  2. Most patients attain sufficient stability to be returned to referring doctors and followed in a traditional consultative model, with either:
    a. A community psychiatrist, or
    b. A community internist being the primary doctor, depending on the relative proportion of psychiatric and medical problems.
  3. Occasional patients will improve in function but enter a relatively unstable phase best managed by their continuing involvement with a subspecialized medical-psychiatric program at a referral center.
F. Medical-psychiatric units are rapidly developing at:
  1. Tertiary-care hospitals.
  2. Some community hospitals.
G. Preconditions for developing a unit would include:
  1. An adequate number of psychiatrists with interests in combined problems.
  2. Availability of nursing staff willing to combine medical and psychiatric practice.
  3. Administrative support to meet requirements for DRG exemption.
  4. In community hospitals these units can be operated on an open staff model, provided that adequate medical direction is available to assure the quality of care and the appropriateness of admissions.

V. The Interdisciplinary Geriatric Evaluation/Treatment Program in a Department of Medicine (G. Gottlieb) (Larson, Reifler, Sumi, Canfield, & Chinn, 1985; Reifler & Eisdorfer, 1980; Waxman & Carner, 1984)

A. This program:
  1. Integrates expertise in:
    a. Primary care.

b. Geriatric internal medicine.
  c. Gerontologic nursing.
  d. Geriatric psychiatry.
  e. Social work.
 2. Provides evaluation and care of older adults with a combination of disorders:
    a. Medical.
    b. Neurologic.
    c. Psychiatric.
 3. Features a three-visit interdisciplinary assessment with:
    a. Comprehensive medical and psychiatric examinations completed by functional, environmental, and family evaluations.
    b. Neurological and neuropsychological assessment of patients with evidence of cognitive impairment.
    c. Simultaneous psychiatric and medical intervention.
B. Important advantages are that:
 1. Access to psychiatric care is routine and therefore not limited by stigma.
 2. Family stresses are addressed immediately, and individual and family resources are identified and nurtured.
 3. Primary-care providers, including psychiatrists in private and community-based practice, are provided with:
    a. Access to technologies, assessment, and multidisciplinary expertise.
    b. An extensive data base.
    c. Better access to family and community resources.
    d. A recommended (or, if desired, implemented) treatment plan.
    e. Rapid and convenient referral without the risk of losing patients to other providers.
    f. Reinforcement of the primacy of the referring physician, since most treatment strategies rely upon the skills of the primary provider for implementation.
C. The goals of the program are:
 1. Primarily evaluation and consultation.
 2. Secondarily to offer ongoing primary care if requested.
 3. Also to be a community link for caregivers and families of progressively impaired individuals.
D. The main principles of treatment are:
 1. Optimization of overall function.
 2. Health promotion.
 3. Conservatism in appropriate pharmacologic management.
E. Suitable patients are those with:
 1. Progressive cognitive impairment.

2. Subtle or treatment-resistant psychiatric disorder.
3. Complex medical presentations.
4. Suspected cognitive or emotional disorders associated with medical or iatrogenic etiologies.
5. Combined medical-psychiatric disorders in acutely ill patients and in individuals with chronic disability.

F. This model of treatment, involving collaboration with geriatricians, nurses, and social workers, can be generalized to:
   1. Psychiatrists with special training or interest in geriatrics.
   2. An individual provider's practice, on a smaller scale, profitably, and without dominating the practice.

VI. Hospital-Based Psychiatric Ambulatory Care and Outreach (J. Barsa)
(Barsa, Kass, Beels, Gurland, & Charles, 1985)

A. A geriatric psychiatrist can enter a general adult psychiatry clinic that has no geriatric psychiatry program and influence the clinic to build a multifaceted geropsychiatry service without spending a lot of money or using extra facility space.
   1. The service director can piece together a salary with partial funding through:
      a. A psychiatry fellowship.
      b. A state or city service line.
      c. A grant from a university center for geriatrics.
   2. Within the clinic, the geriatric psychiatrist needs to:
      a. Launch initiatives that establish a presence as a role model.
      b. Change methods of service delivery to maximize service reimbursement (e.g., initiate a group therapy program).
      c. Convince trainees and permanent staff to voluntarily expand their patient load to allow more treatment for senior citizens.
      d. Organize special geropsychiatry lectures and supervision.
      e. Custom design geriatric mental health projects for clinic trainees and permanent staff to meet their special goals in the mental health field. For example, a nurse with a special interest in community outreach can be encouraged to help form a mental health outreach project in a senior citizens' housing program.
   3. Even with a well-established clinic program, senior citizens may resist attending the psychiatry clinic. Therefore, three types of offsite geriatric psychiatry programs are needed.
      a. Geropsychiatric consultation to medical/surgical clinics within the hospital setting.

(1) Supplementation of a consultation liaison psychiatry presence in the medical clinic can be achieved by stationing a geropsychiatric or a psychiatric fellow in the medical site. Rather than simply providing consultations, the psychiatrist runs a "clinic within a clinic," giving mental health treatments to seniors in the medical clinic. This bypasses some of the stigma associated with elderly people's coming to psychiatry clinics.
(2) A psychiatric fellow can lead geriatric discussion groups with the head nurses in the medical-surgical clinics.
b. Geropsychiatric consultations to senior citizens' centers. Cooperating permanent staff (nurses, psychologists, social workers, and public psychiatry fellows), using their discretionary time, go to various senior centers and offer individual and group therapy at those sites. Since the centers are places where the seniors feel comfortable, they readily accept the mental health services.
c. Geropsychiatric home screening can be accomplished by linking up with the state-run mobile geriatrics team. This team often lacks a geriatric psychiatrist and appreciates this link.
d. In addition, it is important to coordinate the consultation service with:
(1) Other area agencies.
(2) Inpatient care facilities.
(3) Research units, in order to avoid a duplication of services.

VII. The Psychiatrist's Role in Linking Community Services (C. Cohen)
(Cohen & Briggs, 1976)

A. Over the past two decades there has been a dramatic expansion in the number of community social service agencies serving inner-city aging populations.
1. Such agencies often develop around senior lunch programs, outreach programs, health services, or socialization activities.
2. As these programs expand, staff become more cognizant of the degree of psychological distress among their client population.
3. These agencies identify a need for direct psychiatric treatment as well as for staff supervision in dealing with the psychosocial issues of their clients.
4. In some cases the initial request for services comes from the agency; in other instances it arises from an institution or individual practitioner.

5. A majority of these agencies lack adequate funds, and alternative methods for supporting a psychiatrist have to be explored.
B. The potential funding for supporting a psychiatrist to fill this gap can come from several principal sources.
   1. A university medical center training program that hopes to provide a broader clinical experience for its psychiatric trainees.
   2. A university-based program that plans to expand its research into community problems.
   3. A university-based program that views community service as part of its mission.
   4. An individual psychiatrist who wishes to supplement his or her income through Medicaid/Medicare reimbursement.
C. In order to ensure the continuation of the psychiatric services, they must win recognition of their usefulness from the sources of support.
   1. For university-based programs this may occur when:
      a. Trainees report positive feedback from the experience.
      b. Research data are published.
      c. Grants are generated.
      d. The university receives media coverage and public accolades for the services.
      e. Mechanisms are developed for receiving Medicaid/Medicare reimbursement for the clinical services.
   2. Once a clinical population is identified, government programs (e.g., Community Support Services Program in New York State) can sometimes be used to pay for clinical staff services.
   3. For the individual private practitioner the decision to continue services will ultimately depend on whether adequate income is generated. In such instances, should the original psychiatrist depart, the possibility of recruiting a new psychiatrist is markedly enhanced because of the availability of patients to begin a practice.

VIII. The Psychiatrist and the Nursing Home (P. Birkett) (Rovner, Kafonek, Filipp, Lucas, & Folstein, 1986; Sabin, Vitug, & Mark, 1982)

A. There is a pressing need for mental health services in nursing homes.
   1. The need exists because:
      a. The decline in the population of state mental hospitals in the United States has been paralleled by a growth in the popula-

tion of nursing homes. It has been suggested that the so-called deinstitutionalization of the mentally disordered is a reinstitutionalization of this population in nursing homes instead of mental hospitals.
   b. Surveys of mental illness in nursing homes reveal a predominance of mental disorder. About 30% to 80% of the nursing home population suffer from major psychiatric illness, such as dementia and depression.
   c. Adjustment disorders with depressed mood also occur among the minority of patients who are not demented but who suffer from a specific disabling physical condition.
   d. Admission diagnoses are usually of physical conditions and thus obscure the mix of psychiatric, medical, and social factors that lead to institutionalization in a nursing home.
2. Not all institutions for the elderly are nursing homes, and it is important for the psychiatrist dealing with an institution to be aware of its official category and the level of resources that pertain. Some of the types of institutions are:
   a. Skilled nursing facilities.
   b. Health-related facilities.
   c. Adult care homes.
   d. Single-room-occupancy hotels.
   e. Group homes.
3. Skilled nursing facilities are:
   a. Staffed by registered nurses.
   b. Capable of a considerable amount of sophisticated medical skills short of intravenous infusions or surgery.
   c. Limited in their psychiatric abilities; for example, they cannot (with the exception of California) lock doors to keep patients in.
   d. Able to employ psychiatrists as:
      (1) Consultants, either on a private fee-for-service basis or as part of a publicly funded service.
      (2) Primary-care physicians.
      (3) Administrators.
B. In certain ways the private consultation at a nursing home resembles a general hospital consultation.
   1. However, it also has its special demands.
      a. It is often necessary to visit the nursing home; psychiatrists who are willing to do so will find themselves in demand, since these patients are not very portable.
      b. It will often be found that administrators or nursing staff rather than the attending physician of record have requested

the consultation, and the first step may often have to be a discussion with them as to the reason for consultation.
   c. It will sometimes be found that psychiatric assessment is necessary to satisfy Medicaid requirements for documentation [e.g., in New York, RUGs (resource utilization groups) forms are required].
   d. Contact with the family should be made when possible but is not always easy. A major socioeconomic factor leading to nursing home placement is the fact that daughters or daughters-in-law work.
   e. Questions of payment may have to be discussed at an early stage. The psychiatrist should be aware of the variable and usually inadequate provision made by Medicare.
2. A psychiatrist working at a nursing home, even in a consultative role, assumes a responsibility for some aspects of the standards of care.
   a. Although dementia is seldom in itself a cause for requesting consultation, the consultant should
      (1) Place on record a quantified assessment of the degree of dementia present.
      (2) Ascertain whether an adequate workup for treatable causes of dementia or delirium has been done, with particular reference to the possibility of overmedication's contributing to cognitive dysfunction.
   b. Depression and behavioral disorders are common causes for requesting consultation. If psychotropic medication is recommended, the family should be made aware of the nature and side effects of the agent prescribed and reassured that tranquilizers are not being overused.
   c. Sometimes referrals are made with the hope that the patient can be transferred to another setting; this may lead to difficulties presented by a fragmented system of care.
      (1) Psychiatry patients with concomitant physical complaints are sometimes unacceptable to many psychiatric units.
      (2) There may be ethical and legal problems in getting a demented patient to sign for informal admission to a general hospital unit.
      (3) State-funded facilities will often refuse to accept behaviorally disturbed and demented patients from nursing homes.
      (4) When there is a recommendation for hospitalization and it cannot be accomplished because of inadequate local facilities, it is well to place on record in writing that

adequate application has been made and that the difficulty arises from causes outside the consultant psychiatrist's control.
    d. In many cases the psychiatrist consults to a nursing home as a representative of a publicly funded agency.
        (1) In such cases he or she will also have to ascertain, preferably in writing, the policies of the agency.
        (2) The organizational allegiance must be clear if the referral is from the nursing home for the purpose of hospitalization and the psychiatrist is sent by a state agency whose policy is to avoid hospitalization.
3. The psychiatrist in the nursing home who functions also as a primary-care physician is, by virtue of his/her dual role, able to:
    a. Reduce the administration of multiple medications.
    b. Recognize more accurately physical symptoms based on depression.
    c. Use psychotropic medications more appropriately.
    d. Lower the frequency of sedation and adverse drug effects, physical morbidity, and mortality.
4. Under federal law it is necessary for each nursing home to have a medical director.
    a. Since some nursing homes are often close to being like miniature mental hospitals, psychiatry is an appropriate specialty for the medical director.
    b. Psychotherapeutic skills may be useful in improving the ability of staff members to deal sensitively with patients and to cope with the strain of the caretaking role.
5. The psychiatrist is likely to play an increasingly active part in the nursing home's organization.
    a. In the United States in 1980, there were already 20,000 nursing homes, housing 1.2 million patients.
    b. The very old (those over age 75), who are at the greatest risk of admission to a nursing home, are the fastest-growing segment of the elderly population.

IX. Linkages Between Service Disciplines in Inpatient Psychiatric Centers (J. Toner)
(Campbell & Vivell, 1985; Toner, 1982)

A. The interdisciplinary treatment team is a key link between service disciplines in inpatient psychiatric settings.
    1. Members of the interdisciplinary team require special training to enable them to work effectively together. Training, which can

be accomplished either formally or informally on the unit, can be:
   a. Directed at facilitating and encouraging a teamlike approach to patient care.
   b. Durable, in that effects last beyond the period of training.
   c. Concentrated on developing team cohesiveness.
   d. Not solely reliant on a single group leader/facilitator.
   e. Based on teaching the team how to continue and maintain self-learning processes.
   2. Because of the high turnover of staff in many psychiatric hospitals, the training program specifically avoids emphasis on:
      a. Didactic methods.
      b. Charismatic leadership.
      c. Individual, as opposed to team, learning.
B. The Program for Organizing Interdisciplinary Self Education (POISE) (Toner, 1982) is one program that has demonstrated that the above principles can be applied successfully in a psychiatric hospital.
   1. The learning process covers:
      a. Skills.
      b. Knowledge.
      c. Attitudes toward:
         (1) The role each member of the team plays in assessing the patient.
         (2) Linking each member's assessment to a treatment plan.
         (3) Systematic approaches and procedures for making appropriate treatment decisions. The treatment decision guide, a guide designed by the interdisciplinary team members specifically for patient management in their particular institution, provides a key to arriving at available treatment alternatives in that institution.
   2. After interdisciplinary treatment team members are trained by a facilitator to develop their idiosyncratic treatment decision guide, the guide provides a crucial device by which team members relate to one another in operating the ongoing system themselves.
   3. To further the ongoing self-learning process, the systematic learning methods are also applied by the team to:
      a. Surveys of specific needs for treatment of the elderly patient population in the psychiatric hospital.
      b. Refinement of criteria for specific discharge dispositions of elderly patients.
      c. Quality controls of treatment and its outcome.

X. The Need for Linkages Between the Public and Private Sectors (B. Meyers)
(Keill, 1986; Stein, 1983)

A. The organization of the components of the geriatric mental health care delivery system must be embedded in the context of the two sources of service and reimbursement: the public and private sectors.
   1. The dual (public and private) health care systems in this country:
      a. Provide opportunities for greater comprehensiveness of care.
      b. Present potential obstacles to a truly integrated and continuous approach.
      c. Necessitate the establishment of linkages between public and private sectors to prevent the creation of more and larger cracks into which the elderly psychiatric patient can unfortunately fall.
   2. The functioning of the components of an organized mental health service will be substantially influenced by:
      a. The sector to which they belong.
      b. The relevance of the sector's financial nature to the existence of the particular service.
      c. The accessibility of the component service to patients from another financial sector.
      d. The feasibility of creating linkages with services from the other sector.
   3. A review of major components presently in place and existing linkages demonstrates the following:
      a. When care is conceptualized on a continuum between inpatient and office treatment, a greater number of resources are available in the public sector. The statement applies to types of resources as well as absolute numbers; day hospitals, day treatment programs, and mobile geriatric teams rarely exist in the private sector.
      b. The increased options and different levels of care within the public sector allow for greater vertical integration and continuity of care within this sector.
      c. Despite its increased comprehensiveness and continuity, the public sector has less psychiatric manpower and must rely heavily on the nonmedical mental health professional and the multidisciplinary team. This "spreading thin" of psychiatric manpower within the public sector is especially disconcerting in regard to the care of the medically fragile elderly with mental health problems.

d. The majority of psychiatric hospital beds are in the private sector, and similarly, a preponderance of psychiatrists are private practitioners.
e. There are difficulties with the current policy on reimbursement.
   (1) There was a $250 annual outpatient ceiling for Medicare reimbursement, which was recently increased, to psychiatrists. Medicare's reimbursement for inpatient treatment is more equitable but severely restricts outpatient reimbursement.
   (2) The reimbursement pattern seriously undermines continuity of care within the private sector and can lead to:
      (a) Premature and unnecessary psychiatric hospitalization, perhaps explaining why 85% of geriatric mental health care is provided on an inpatient basis (Gatz, Smyer, & Lawton, 1980).
      (b) Patients moving between private inpatient treatment and postdischarge care in public clinics.
      (c) Pressure for mental health treatment by nonpsychiatric physicians in ambulatory settings.
f. Most elderly residents of nursing homes suffer emotional difficulties, and their needs are not adequately addressed by either sector.
g. A growth in academic centers.
   (1) The burgeoning knowledge about geriatric psychiatry resulting from NIMH-supported research and training has created academic centers capable of providing excellence in clinical care and education.
   (2) A gap exists between these knowledge banks and the preponderance of practitioners.
   (3) The problem is presumably more severe in the private sector because of the absence of integrated systems to assure quality of training and quality of care.
2. The extent to which the public and private sectors are "separate but equal" versus a two-tier system with differences in quality is undetermined. Nevertheless, a number of suggestions can improve care within the current two-system context:
   a. Continuity of care between levels and components of each system must be facilitated.
   b. Intersystem networking should be expedited
      (1) to facilitate patient access to components of both systems.
      (2) to minimize loss of continuity of care.
   c. Regulations are needed that foster continuity of care between

inpatient and outpatient settings to increase psychiatric service to nursing homes and to disseminate clinical knowledge from the academic centers to the practicing clinicians.
   d. In assessing the nature, feasibility, and accessibility of any psychogeriatric service, its location within the public-private sector matrix needs to be determined and the possibility of creating linkages with appropriate components from the other sector determined.

XI. Social Services for the Aged (A. Monk) (Steinberg, 1985; Tobin & Toseland, 1985)

A. Social services for older persons have evolved in the United States without the benefit of thought-out blueprints. They resulted instead from expedient reactions to public clamor and political pressures.
   1. Over the years, more than 200 social programs of national scope have been mandated by public policy.
      a. They are best understood as a continuum ranging from services for the well and independent to ones for the severely frail in need of institutionalization.
      b. The sites of service delivery include the home, the community, the hospital, and the long-term care facility.
      c. The services enhance or compensate for waning functional, cognitive, perceptual, affective, and social competencies.
   2. Policy analysts and planners are primarily concerned with how well the service system addresses the manifest needs of the elderly and how accessible it is to them.
      a. Older persons need more than one service at any given time.
      b. Different providers attend to separate eligibility requirements.
      c. For 30 years the Social Security Act provided an income rather than a service strategy toward the aged.
      d. The Older Americans Act was introduced to foster the coordination of services and the development of gap-filling new services.
   3. Service integration is fostered at the local level through more than 600 Area Agencies on Aging.
      a. Some are coterminous with a single city or county, and others may cover an entire state.
      b. They favor:
         (1) Single points of entry.
         (2) Up-to-date information and referral.
         (3) The assurance of a true continuum of care.

c. They coordinate services over which they may not have statutory authority.
d. Some do not directly provide any major program other than nutrition programs.
e. They rely primarily on negotiation with other public and voluntary agencies.
4. A separate approach to service coordination evolved from case-management experiences.
a. These have been tested by "channeling grants" fostered by the Health Care Administration over the past decade.
b. Case management organizes an individualized package of case-related services.
c. Case managers:
(1) Assess the problems and needs of applicants.
(2) Determine the range of required interventions.
(3) Consult with a multidisciplinary team of providers.
(4) Negotiate and advocate with agencies to ensure that service will be delivered as scheduled.
(5) Monitor and reassess the condition of the beneficiary.
d. Case management is the inevitable corollary of an age of specialization.
(1) People in need and, most specifically, frail older persons find it difficult to negotiate and obtain the services they may be entitled to.
(2) Case management is a service that facilitates both access and the assurance of obtaining other services. It cannot, however, create needed services when they do not exist.
5. The fine-tuning of existing services and creation of much-needed new services will continue as long as life expectancy and the numbers of older persons keep increasing.

XII. Informal Family Care (L. Grau)

A. The majority of older people with debilitating physical and mental disorders reside in the community rather than in institutions.
1. Therefore, families:
a. Assume major responsibility for procuring and coordinating formal services and care such as that provided by:
(1) Psychiatrists or other mental health workers.
(2) Primary-care physicians.
(3) Professional and nonprofessional homecare workers.
b. Often provide direct care, including:

(1) Personal care.
(2) Instrumental assistance.
B. The Elderly Person's Caretakers.
1. The primary informal caretaker is most likely to be:
a. The spouse.
b. A child (most often a daughter or daughter-in-law) when there is no spouse or the spouse is very frail.
2. Secondary informal caretaker(s) may be other family members, friends, and neighbors.
3. Family caretaking:
a. May be superior to institutional care.
b. May be a substantial burden for individual family caretakers and the family unit:
(1) The stress of round-the-clock caretaking can result in depression and anxiety.
(2) The caretakers are often limited in their ability to engage in work and social activities outside the home, leading to social isolation and potential economic hardship.
C. Major problems in the community care of the elderly mentally ill include:
1. There is a lack of public programs that focus on the mental health needs of the elderly persons and their family caretakers.
2. Medicare coverage for outpatient psychiatric care, although increased in 1988, is still quite limited.
3. Medicare does not cover services such as respite and day care.
4. Medicaid services and eligibility criteria vary widely from state to state; they are generally limited with respect to mental health services and programs.
5. There are inadequate numbers of mental health workers with training and experience in geriatric mental health.
6. Diagnosis and treatment often become the responsibility of physicians, who may be unaware or uncertain about the various and complex expressions of organic and psychiatric mental disorders among the elderly.

XIII. The British National Health Service as a System of Care (J. Copeland)

A. The development of services in Britain had the undoubted advantage of a nationwide General Practitioner (GP) Primary Care Service.
1. Evidence for this is seen in the facts that
a. Nearly all residents, even those who elect for private care, are registered with a general practitioner.

b. The primary-care team coordinates the patient's treatment.
c. GPs treat the vast majority of psychiatric illness, referring fewer than 1 in 10 cases to a specialist.
d. They are paid a higher per capita fee for patients aged 65 and over.
e. The GP may request the consultant to assess the patient in his/her own home. The consultant receives an extra payment for this service.

2. Consultants in the Psychiatry of Old Age
    a. The psychiatric consultants and junior medical staffs are on fixed salaries.
    b. Districts are increasingly served by a consultant in the psychiatry of old age.
    c. The Royal College of Psychiatrists has laid down strict rules for the training of those junior hospital doctors who wish to become consultants.
    d. The psychogeriatricians or consultants in the psychiatry of old age have tended to keep their limited resources for:
        (1) New referrals aged 65 and over.
        (2) Longstanding outpatients as the patients' age advances.
        (3) All elderly patients with both functional and organic illnesses.
    e. In some districts, the psychogeriatrician and geriatrician:
        (1) Admit patients to each other's hospital beds.
        (2) Do joint ward rounds.
        (3) Assess patients together.

3. Large mental hospitals are being closed, leading to the growth of psychogeriatric units in general hospitals. These consist of:
    a. Inpatient beds.
    b. A day hospital.
    c. Long-stay accommodation.
    d. The hospital team consists of:
        (1) Consultant, who acts as the leader.
        (2) Nurse.
        (3) Clinical psychologist.
        (4) Social worker.

4. One of the most important developments in British psychiatry of recent years has been the establishment of community psychiatric nurses.
    a. These are senior nurses with psychiatric qualifications.
    b. They work full-time in the community but are attached to the hospital team or, occasionally, to the general practitioner.
    c. They regularly visit patients in their homes.

d. They ensure that medication is taken.
e. They give advice to caring relatives and monitor the burden of care.
f. They follow up on patients who do not keep appointments.
g. They coordinate the GP and the consultant service.
5. The Royal College of Psychiatrists has recommended that for a population of 100,000 persons, assuming 15% aged over 65, there should be:
a. 15 acute beds staffed by 12.5 nurses.
b. 45 aftercare beds requiring 30 nurses.
c. 30 daycare/day treatment places with 6 nurses.
d. 2 community-based psychiatric nurses.
e. 1 consultant psychogeriatrician.
f. An administrative secretary.
g. A clinical psychologist (half-time).
h. A senior occupational therapist (half-time) and a basic grade occupational therapist (half time), with one full-time and one half-time aide.
i. A senior or basic grade physiotherapist (three-quarter time) and 1 aide.
j. Access to speech therapy.
6. If the National Health Service is valuable, it is partly because of the coordination it achieves in health care.

REFERENCES

Barsa, J., Kass, F., Beels, C., Gurland, B., & Charles, E. (1985). Development of a cost-efficient psychogeriatrics service. *The American Journal of Psychiatry, 142*(2), 238-241.

Campbell, L. J., & Vivell, S. (1985). *Interdisciplinary team training for primary care in geriatrics: An educational model for programs* (No. 585-586). Washington, DC: U.S. Government Printing Office.

Cohen, C. I., & Briggs, F. (1976). A small storefront clinic on the Bowery. *Journal of Studies in Alcohol, 37,* 1336-1340.

Finkel, S. I. (1983). Mental health services for the elderly: Current policies and future directions. *The Psychiatric Hospital, 14,* 76-81.

Fogel, B., & Stoudemire, A. (1986). Organization and development of medical/psychiatric units: Part II. *Psychosomatics, 27,* 417-426.

Gatz, M., Smyer, M. A., & Lawton, M. P. (1980). The mental health system and the older adult. In L. W. Poon (Ed.), *Aging in the 1980's: Psychological issues* (pp. 5-18). Washington, DC: American Psychological Association.

German, P. S., Shapiro, S., & Skinner, E. A. (1985). Mental health of the elderly: Use of health and mental health services. *Journal of the American Geriatrics Society, 33,* 246-252.

Hargreaves, W. A. (1986). Theory of psychiatric treatment systems: An approach. *Arch Gen Psychiatry, 43,* 701-705.

Keill, S. L. (1986). Integration of psychiatric services into a comprehensive health care system for the aged. *Bulletin of the New York Academy of Medicine, 62,* 182-187.

Larson, E. B., Reifler, B. V., Sumi, S. M., Canfield, C. G., & Chinn, N. M. (1985). Diagnostic evaluation of 200 elderly outpatients with suspected dementia. *Journal of Gerontology, 40,* 536-543.

Reifler, B. V., & Eisdorfer, C. A. (1980). A clinic for the impaired elderly and their families. *American Journal of Psychiatry, 137,* 1399-1403.

Rovner, B. W., Kafonek, S., Filipp, L., Lucas, M., & Folstein, M. (1986). Prevalence of mental illness in a common nursing home. *American Journal of Psychiatry, 143,* 1446-1449.

Sabin, T. D., Vitug, A. J., & Mark, V. H. (1982). Are nursing home diagnoses and treatment inadequate? *Journal of the American Medical Association, 248,* 321-322.

Stein, E. M. (1983). Treating the aged: How the public system affects the private system. *The Psychiatric Hospital, 14,* 82-86.

Steinberg, R. M. (1985). Access assistance and case management. In A. Monk (Ed.), *Handbook of gerontological services* (pp. 109-141). New York: Van Nostrand Reinhold.

Stoudemire, A., & Fogel, B. (1986). Organization and development of combined medical/psychiatric units: Part I. *Psychosomatics, 27,* 341-345.

Targum, S. D., & Docherty, J. P. (1985). The future of research in private psychiatric hospitals. *The Psychiatric Hospital, 16,* 115-119.

Tobin, S. S., & Toseland, R. (1985). Models of services for the elderly. In A. Monk (Ed.), *Handbook of gerontological services* (pp. 549-567). New York: Van Nostrand Reinhold.

Toner, J. (1982). Interdisciplinary treatment team training: A training program in geriatric assessment for health care providers. In C. K. Nicholson & J. I. Nicholson (Eds.), *The personalized care model for the elderly* (2nd ed.) (pp. 25-37). New York: Nicholson and Nicholson.

Waxman, H. M., & Carner, E. A. (1984). Physicians' recognition, diagnosis, and treatment of mental disorders in elderly medical patients. *The Gerontologist, 24,* 593-597.

11

Legal Issues in Geriatric Psychiatry

F. M. Baker and Sanford I. Finkel

INTRODUCTION

The legal issues arising in the clinical care of older patients are discussed. Beginning with an overview of general principles and definitions, specific topics are addressed, including wills, civil contracts, guardianship/conservatorship, and competence with respect to specific legal issues. Included within the specific legal issues are the hopelessly ill patient and the living-will legislation.

I. General Principles Regarding Legal Issues (Meisel, Roth, & Lidz, 1977; Bell, Schmidt, & Miller, 1981; Appelbaum & Roth, 1981; Baker, Perr, & Yesavage, 1986)

- A. The specific legal issue being addressed may or may not be stated clearly. The first task is to clarify the specific legal issue(s) being addressed.
- B. The core aspect of any legal decision involving an older person, for example, commitment, consent, or civil law, centers on the issue of competency.
- C. Competence is not a single concept. It is defined by law and relates to the specific issue at hand, for example, competence to refuse treatment.
- D. In *de jure* competence persons are competent due to their status under the law, that is, all adults are presumed to be competent for a

variety of purposes unless found incompetent for a specific purpose. Depending on the jurisdiction (location within the United States), children and adolescents up to a certain age by the definition of the law (*de jure*) are incompetent: unable to make contracts, marry, or decide various aspects of their medical care. An example of a jurisdictional exception: a person aged 13 or older can consent to treatment for drug abuse by Texas state statute.
- E. If an adult is in fact incompetent, this is termed *de facto* incompetency.
- F. The psychiatric assessment performed to address a specific legal issue actually gathers information that enables the psychiatrist to form an opinion whether in fact (*de facto*) the patient is competent or incompetent for a specific purpose.
- G. Factors considered in this psychiatric assessment include:
    1. The cognitive capacity of the individual.
    2. The ability of the individual to make decisions.
    3. The individual's judgment as applied to the particular issue at hand.
- H. From the viewpoint of the law, *de facto* incompetence does not exist. The *de facto* opinion of the psychiatrist is presented as data in a competency hearing that contributes to addressing, by the judge, the *de jure* issues at hand.

II. Testimonial Capacity
(Perr, 1981; Sadoff, 1975)

- A. Definition: the capacity to testify in court requires that the individual:
    1. Is able to recount factual data.
    2. Understands the nature of swearing under oath.
- B. By law, a judge is given the authority to screen individuals concerning their capacity to testify.
- C. The ability of all persons to recollect significant data over time varies. Due to the long delay before a case reaches court (sometimes several years), any person who has developed a memory disorder may no longer be a reliable informant.

III. Testamentary Capacity

- A. Definition: the capacity to make a will requires:
    1. Knowledge that one is making a will.
    2. Knowledge of the extent of the property involved (nature of his/her bounty).

3. Knowledge of the likely heirs ("natural" recipients) and their relationship to the individual.
B. Some jurisdictions may require, also, that the individual have the ability to communicate such desires.
C. Although advanced age does not preclude making a will, it may raise the issue of competency due to ageism.
D. Undue influence: although a person may have testamentary capacity at the time of the signing of the will, the person's state of mind may be such that he/she could be unduly influenced (manipulated) by a conniving, controlling individual or by a person with whom he/she has a trusting relationship based on that person's professional status (fiduciary relationship).
   1. Undue influence implies:
      a. A weakness or disability on the part of the person making the will (a psychiatric opinion).
      b. Suspicious circumstances involved in the making of the will (a judicial determination).
E. Lucid interval: in a person with varying cognitive states, a period may occur during which the person has the temporary capacity to make a will, that is, "a lucid interval." Repeat mental-status examinations at different times of day serve to document the presence or absence of fluctuations in the person's cognitive state, whether caused by illness, medication, changing environmental stress, or other factors.
F. If a person makes a partial subsequent will or addition, termed a codicil, the validity of the codicil may be questioned.
G. Many attorneys request a concurrent psychiatric examination at the time that a will is made by an elderly person whose testamentary capacity may be questioned. Some psychiatrists instruct their patients to see them on a day a change in a will is made.
H. Wills may be challenged in the following circumstances:
   1. A later will differs from an earlier will (any will acts to revoke prior wills) and different relatives may benefit by one, rather than the other, will.
   2. The older person disposes of his/her property, his/her assets in a way that is "detrimental" to family members who expect the property/assets to be left to them.
   3. The older person marries or becomes involved, affectionately, with a person of whom family members do not approve.
   4. Before a will is made, the older person becomes mentally incapacitated.
   5. Before a will is made, the older person becomes physically incapacitated.

6. The older person becomes more susceptible to the influence of others.
   7. The older person refuses a medical intervention or procedure that may be necessary to prolong his/her life.
I. Marriage is a civil contract.
   1. The marriage of an elderly person to a younger companion may cause distress to the children of an earlier marriage, for example, the "Groucho Marx" situation or the "Trixie" syndrome.
   2. Contesting the marriage contract requires proving that the elderly person did not understand the circumstances and meaning of the marital agreement.
   3. In general, courts do not readily invalidate a marriage.
   4. If the state statutes include no-fault divorce, termination of a marital contract is less of an issue as neither participant needs to assign blame.
J. Custody disputes may arise for the elderly if the parents of a deceased spouse (the grandparents of the child) are in conflict with the surviving spouse. Specific issues involved here are:
   1. The competency of the grandparents for parenting.
   2. The best overall environment for the child.

IV. Guardianship
(Perr, 1981; Sadoff, 1975)

A. Definition: under the Uniform Probate Code, guardianship refers to control over a person.
B. If a state has *not* adopted the Uniform Probate Code, then the definition of a guardian can vary.
C. Guardianship differs from conservatorship in that guardianship does not permit involuntary hospitalization for psychiatric treatment.
D. If a state has not adopted the Uniform Probate Code and the state statute unifies guardianship over both the person and his/her property, the guardian can by law:
   1. Provide for medical care.
   2. Volunteer the patient for hospitalization and treatment (bypassing the need for commitment).
   3. Note: relatives have challenged such a unified statute.
E. Decisions of a guardian include:
   1. Making medical decisions and granting consent for medical treatment or procedures.
   2. Deciding the place of abode, such as a nursing home.
   3. Admitting the person to a hospital.

F. Under the Uniform Probate Code, memory impairment or physical deterioration are not a sufficient basis for the judgment of "incapacity"; there must be a clear lack of understanding and ability to communicate.
G. Some states, for example, New Hampshire, focus on a broader, nondiagnostic or therapeutic approach that emphasizes specific acts or occurrences of incapacity or functional limitation. Specific data from the functional assessment (Nolan, 1984) may be required as part of the guardianship proceedings; this functional assessment may include determination of the individual's income adequacy and spending pattern, adequacy of food, clothing, and the ability to eat, choice of diet, ability to dress and undress, sensory functioning, and physical functioning including the ability to talk, climb stairs, reach, bend, get in and out of chair and tub, and other functions. The functional assessment may be performed by a physician or a nurse.
H. The standard for guardianship varies by state, and it is important to know the standard of your state. While the Uniform Probate Code emphasizes lack of cognitive and communicative ability as a necessary criterion for incompetence, several states have added the requirement for some objectively observable behavior as evidence of incapacity. Some states, for example, Ohio, require a diagnosis of the *cause* of the socially disapproved behavior that may necessitate guardianship.
I. Recent state laws have required:
  1. A functional evaluation to be made.
  2. That it present specific documentation of behaviors of incapacity or functional limitations within six months of the filing date.
  3. That at least one act of improper care of self or property has occurred within 20 days of filing.

V. Conservatorship
(Perr, 1981; Sadoff, 1975)

A. Definition: under the Uniform Probate Code, conservatorship refers to the right of control over another person's property and/or person, as adjudicated by a court of law.
B. In some states without a Uniform Probate Code, the distinction between guardianship and conservatorship is confused, reversed, or reflects overlapping powers.
C. Responsibilities of the conservatorship include:
  1. Responsibility for property of the person.
  2. The ability to contract on behalf of the person, for example,

contracts for personal care (nursing home or medical care contract).
D. Removal of conservatorship and guardianship requires that the older person demonstrate that he/she is no longer incompetent. This may prove to be a more difficult procedure than the initial legal proceedings that found the individual incompetent.
1. It usually means demonstration of improvement in physical and/or mental condition.

VI. Competence with Respect to Specific Legal Issues

A. Hospitalization (Perr, 1978a; Tibbles, 1978; Addington v. Texas, 1979)
1. Occurs voluntarily if:
  a. The person knows the nature and purpose of hospitalization.
  b. The person accepts the fact either of illness or the need for evaluation or care.
  c. The person is, in general, cooperative with the proposed plan of hospitalization.
2. Hospitalization occurs voluntarily in a mildly impaired older patient if:
  a. The patient assents by his/her behavior.
  b. There is no conflict between family, patient, and caregivers.
3. In the older patient with significant impairment:
  a. The next-of-kin should be advised of the need for hospitalization.
  b. Whether or not the nearest of kin (spouse or adult child) can assent to the relative's hospitalization varies by state.
4. Involuntary hospitalization, again depending on the jurisdiction, is governed by one of two principles.
  a. The police powers principle, which considers the dangerousness of the person to him- or herself or others. The state has an interest in maintaining the public safety and will use *police power* to restrict the freedom of persons judged dangerous. In Lessard v. Schmidt (1972) the U.S. Supreme Court defined dangerousness as "an extreme likelihood that if the person is not confined, he will do immediate harm to himself or others." The Court also defined *imminent danger* as "based at minimum on a recent act, attempt, or threat to do substantial harm." In some states, the issue of potential deterioration or progression may be utilized to postulate dangerousness to self or inability to care for oneself for ordinary purposes (e.g., shelter, food, management of physical illness).

b. The *parens patriae* principle, in which the state acts in a paternal parental role to care for people who are mentally disabled and unable to care for themselves. Here, the persons are incompetent due to their inability to make decisions to care for or to manage their needs. In some states such a person is termed gravely disabled in the state statute, and this is the criterion for involuntary hospitalization.
5. Involuntary hospitalization of an older parent by his or her children is viewed with caution by many courts because of:
   a. A past history of claims of abuse due to the tendency of the court to go along with the needs of the adult child (children).
   b. Abuses based on motivations other than the necessary care of the impaired elder.
6. The standard for involuntary hospitalization established by the United States Supreme Court in Addington v. Texas (1979) is "clear and convincing evidence of the need for involuntary hospitalization." Although an older patient may be maintained outside of an institutional setting with round-the-clock supervision, involuntary hospitalization to treat his or her expanding delusional system would be "the most beneficial alternative"—an essential element of the "least restrictive choice."
   a. Some states (e.g., Missouri) have specifically excluded "disorders such as senility . . . not of an actively psychotic nature" as a basis for commitment.
   b. Other states (e.g., Illinois, which excludes dementia as a reason for commitment) allow involuntary hospitalization on the basis of inability to care for his or her own needs in a way that assures survival. In this case, the person is so gravely impaired in his or her functioning that involuntary hospitalization is indicated.
B. Consent or Refusal of Medical Treatment (Wanzer et al., 1984; President's Commission for the Study of Ethical Problems in Medicine and Biomedical and Behavioral Research, 1983; Stone, 1981)
   1. In general, every human being of adult years and sound mind has a right to determine what shall be done with his or her body (Schloendorff v. Society of New York Hospital).
      a. Exceptions to this rule are determined by:
         (1) Law.
         (2) Regulatory policy.
         (3) Judicial decision.
   2. The wishes of the patient found competent by a judge usually prevail.
      a. Judges have allowed patients whom they considered compe-

tent to die by choice, particularly where the individual was aged, crippled, unable to function and/or deteriorating, and where the prognosis for significant improvement was poor.
3. When an elderly patient refuses treatment:
   a. The psychiatrist should evaluate the patient carefully for depression and cognitive dysfunction.
   b. The psychiatrist should explore fully the patient's rationale for his or her decision.
   c. The judge will use the physician's clinical appraisal with other pertinent data to reach a determination regarding the competence or incompetence of the patient to refuse treatment.
   d. Judges frequently decide these matters on the narrow facts of an individual case so that only a very general guideline of principles relevant to the right to refuse treatment exists.
4. The Living Will or Natural Death (Society for the Right to Die, 1986)
   a. Definition: a written document prepared by a person while mentally competent that specifies the circumstances under which he or she will permit the cessation of extraordinary treatment to prolong life and would allow death in accordance with the natural progression of the person's disease.
      (1) Two witnessing signatures are required, as with a will.
      (2) It can be revoked by:
         (a) Written instrument.
         (b) Spoken word.
         (c) Physical act of cancellation.
      (3) Any person, even if incompetent, can revoke a living will (except in Nevada).
   b. The Society for the Right to Die sponsored the model law that was drafted as the 1978 Legislative Services Project of the Yale Law School.
   c. In various states the legislation is termed either the Living Will Act, Natural Death Act, or Right to Die Statute.
   d. As of 1986, 36 states and the District of Columbia had such legislation. The specific states are: Alabama, Arizona, Arkansas, California, Colorado, Connecticut, Delaware, Florida, Georgia, Idaho, Illinois, Indiana, Iowa, Kansas, Louisiana, Maine, Maryland, Mississippi, Missouri, Montana, New York, New Hampshire, New Mexico, North Carolina, Oklahoma, Oregon, South Carolina, Tennessee, Texas, Utah, Vermont, Virginia, Washington, West Virginia, Wisconsin, and Wyoming.
   e. Immunity for physicians who follow the stated wishes of the

individual, for example, a request that extraordinary means not be used to continue his or her life, is a usual provision of the law.
  f. Recently the Society for the Right to Die has encouraged that the naming of a proxy be included as a specific provision of living-will legislation:
     (1) In the event of sudden incapacitation (comatose state) or becoming incompetent, the patient has designated a proxy who is conversant with the patient's wishes concerning terminal care.
     (2) The proxy can share the patient's views with the treating physicians and with them plan appropriate treatment.
     (3) The designation of a proxy under the living-will legislation and the Durable Power of Attorney Statute (see following), if the statute is expanded to include decisions regarding health care, accomplishes the same objective under different statutes.
5. The durable power of attorney statutes (Society for the Right to Die, 1984), which exist in 50 states, were suggested by the report of the President's Commission for the Study of Ethical Problems in Medicine and Biomedical and Behavioral Research (1984) as an alternative device for making health care decisions on behalf of incompetent patients.
  a. Durable power of attorney statutes were intended, originally, to provide decisions affecting the appointer's property.
  b. Expansion of these statutes to include decisions regarding health care requires further study.
  c. The applicability of the durable power of attorney statutes in making health care decisions on behalf of the principal, as well as decisions concerning property, remains unclear.
  d. Some states have passed legislation concerning property and health care.
     (1) Pennsylvania in 1982 (Pa. Cons. Stat. Ann. §§ 5601-5607) and Colorado in 1983 (Colo. Rev. Stat. § 15-14-501 as amended by L. 83) enacted durable power of attorney statutes that provided "the power" to consent or approve on behalf of the principal any medical or other professional care, counsel, or treatment, but did not specify *termination* of treatment.
     (2) The Uniform Durable Power of Attorney Act of California (Calif. Civil Code 2430-2433) does authorize refusal of life-sustaining treatment on behalf of the appointer if the patient is incompetent, refusal being based upon the

prestated wishes of the patient concerning "any type of treatment or placements that (he/she does) not desire."
6. Resuscitation or "No Code"—The Hopelessly Ill Patient (Wanzer et al., 1984)
   a. Physicians from several medical specialties and medical centers throughout the United States presented a comprehensive review of the specific considerations involved in the treatment of the hopelessly ill patient:
      (1) Presented the specific considerations involved.
      (2) Identified the persons involved in the decision to withhold or withdraw life-sustaining procedures for the hopelessly ill patient.
      (3) Offered guidelines to physicians to facilitate their decision making.
   b. Two important precepts were emphasized:
      (1) The patient's role in decision making was paramount.
      (2) Decreasing aggressive treatment of the hopelessly ill patient when such treatment would only prolong a difficult and uncomfortable process of dying was advised.
   c. Ideal circumstances for the hopelessly ill patient to refuse treatment are:
      (1) Clarity of diagnosis and treatment.
      (2) A skilled and sensitive physician.
      (3) A competent and informed patient may have other factors that affect decision making:
         (a) Disease.
         (b) Pain.
         (c) Drugs.
         (d) Altered mental state.
   d. When the patient is incompetent, Wanzer and colleagues (1984) suggested that a proxy for the patient be involved in decision making (see section on Living Will, above).
      (1) The proxy would have knowledge of the patient's treatment wishes.
      (2) If family, close friends, and physicians are all in accord, the appointment of a proxy may not be necessary.
   e. For patients with mild impairment of competence who are somewhat limited in their ability to initiate activities and communication, the objective of care should be freedom from discomfort. The use of emergency resuscitation and intensive care should be guided by:
      (1) The patient's wishes, if known.
      (2) The wishes of the patient's family.

(3) An assessment of the patient's prospect for improvement.
f. Severely demented persons with a new intercurrent illness who previously have made their wishes known (orally or in writing) may ethically have treatment withheld by their physicians if treatment would serve mainly to prolong the dying process.
   (1) A decision about the handling of an acute illness in such a patient is best made before the onset of the acute illness.
   (2) In the *Dinnerstein* case, a Massachusetts court held that a judicial review was not necessary for a "no-code" order for an irreversibly, terminally ill patient with Alzheimer's disease in the event of cardiac or respiratory failure (Schram, Kane, & Roble, 1978).
7. Quality of Life
   a. Other treatment decisions involving consent have invoked the quality-of-life issue.
      (1) When a patient is in a nonsapient, vegetative state requiring life-support systems and where the outlook indicates that no meaningful benefit from "extraordinary" measures is expected, the hospital committee can decide to discontinue such extraordinary measures (*Quinlan* case in New Jersey, 1976).
      (2) When a patient who has previously expressed a desire for withdrawal of life-support systems should he or she ever be in a vegetative state enters such a state, he or she may be permitted to die (Eichner v. Dillon, 1980).
      (3) When the wishes of a profoundly retarded institutionalized male with irreversible bladder cancer were unknown, the court would not allow the patient's mother to refuse treatment (blood transfusion).
      (4) Principle of substituted consent may be used.
         (a) Guardian is appointed for the purpose of the legal review to present the patient's side to the judge.
         (b) The judge is authorized to decide for the incompetent patient, basing his or her decision upon what the patient, if rational, would decide.
         (c) Here the consenting decision of the judge substitutes for the consent of the patient (Superintendent of Belchertown State School v. Saikewicz, 1977).
   b. Various states and courts may follow different procedures and principles in addressing this issue.
   c. In general, the legal trend is to:

(1) Determine what the person would have wished.
(2) Implement that wish.
8. Electroconvulsive Therapy (Klerman, 1978; Salzman, 1977)
   a. Electroconvulsive therapy (ECT) is often effective in the treatment of major affective disorders.
   b. It may be the treatment of choice for some very depressed older patients, particularly those with multiple medical problems and a deteriorating clinical course (cachectic, delusional) in whom drug-drug interactions may make a psychopharmacological approach problematic.
   c. A patient may refuse ECT if he or she:
      (1) Maintains his or her judgment; the ability to think rationally.
      (2) Maintains the capacity to make a decision about the treatment of ECT.
   d. When the individual's ability to think rationally is compromised, a court hearing for a judicial determination of competency is indicated.
   e. When a person's judgment and decision-making capacity are impaired by illness (e.g., severe depression), the procedure for obtaining ECT will vary by state. Frequently it is a two-stage process.
      (1) Converted status from a voluntary patient to a committed patient.
      (2) Obtained a court order for ECT.
   f. States and courts may weigh these issues differently. Knowledge of your particular state's statutes, the decisions made by your state's courts in the past in similar cases, and consultation with an attorney practicing in your state will provide the background knowledge of your state's approach to this issue.
C. Consent for Research (Appelbaum & Roth, 1982; Stanley, 1983; Melnick, Dubler, & Weisbard, 1984)
   1. It is important to remember that patients with Alzheimer's disease or other dementing illness may be competent in some respects and incompetent in others.
      a. A person incompetent to manage his or her finances may retain the capacity to consent to participate in research.
   2. Further, the commitment of a patient with Alzheimer's disease to a psychiatric facility does not necessarily indicate incompetence in every area of functioning.
      a. Careful assessment for competence regarding decision making about a specific issue is required in patients diagnosed as having a dementing illness.

3. Appelbaum and Roth (1982) conceptualized consent to research in four hierarchical steps:
   a. Evidencing a choice—shown by manifesting consent, expressing positive interest in taking part, or cooperating appropriately in early procedures involved in the study.
   b. Functional understanding of the issues.
   c. Rational manipulation of information.
   d. Appreciation of the nature of the situation:
      (1) Any one of these levels of consent could be used, depending on the specific research design and its policy issues.
4. The issues of consent for research in patients with Alzheimer's disease raise specific issues.
   a. Depending upon how far the patient's illness has progressed, the patient may be aphasic, apraxic, and unable to give informed consent.
   b. The benefits of much of the research in this area are not clear.
   c. The common practice of securing permission of relatives has not been reviewed in several state courts, and there is some question whether it will hold up in court (Kolata, 1982).
5. The designation of a proxy to authorize decisions for future research participation, should the person become incapacitated, has been suggested.
   a. Problem: the results of such a policy would probably be an exceedingly small sample (N) that was biased, that is, persons who designated a proxy could be a special subset of all older persons.
6. The use of a living will was suggested for the patient before his or her development of a dementing illness, rather than the use of a proxy or surrogate.
   a. The living will provides more guidance regarding the patient's wishes.
   b. The living will could be completed early in the course of the dementing illness at a point when the person remained competent to make decisions concerning his or her treatment with extraordinary measures and about participating in research.
7. In 1981, the National Institute on Aging held a national conference that developed suggested guidelines for addressing the ethical and legal issues involved in clinical research in senile dementia of the Alzheimer's type (SDAT) (Melnick, Dubler, Weisbard, et al., 1984).
   a. The guidelines consisted of 10 categories.

b. Regarding the guideline pertaining to "Determination of Particular Subject's Capacity for a Specific Protocol," the authors state:
    (1) "The determination of the subject's capacity to consent to participate in research should not be dependent upon an assessment of the subject's overall state of competency" (p. 533).
8. If a patient is judged to be of questionable competence on clinical examination, Stanley (1983) suggested specific efforts to alter the consent process prior to making a determination of incompetence by a hearing:
    a. Making the consent material more readable.
    b. Tailoring the consent information to the needs of the patient as suggested in the preamble of the federal regulation for research with humans (U.S. Department of Health and Human Services, 1981).
    c. Allowing patients to review the consent material for a lengthier time prior to the assessment of competence.
    d. Using teaching and review methods coupled with testing.
    e. Developing rapport that promotes the patients' confidence in the investigator and enables them to ask as many questions as needed.
    f. Involving the patient's family members in the consent process. Relatives may use language more familiar to the patient, thus making the issues regarding consent to research more understandable.

REFERENCES

Addington v. Texas, 441 U.S. 419 (1979).
Appelbaum, P. S., & Roth, L. H. (1981). Clinical issues in the assessment of competence. *Am J Psychiatry, 138*, 1462–1467.
Appelbaum, P. S., & Roth, L. H. (1982). Competency to consent to research. *Arch Gen Psychiatry, 39*, 951–958.
Baker, F. M., Perr, I. N., & Yesavage, J. A. (1986). *Task force report—An overview of legal issues in geriatric psychiatry.* Washington, DC: American Psychiatric Association.
Bell, W. G., Schmidt, W., & Miller, K. (1981). Public guardianship and the elderly: Findings from a national study. *The Gerontologist, 21*, 194–202.
California Durable Power of Attorney for Health Care. Calif. Civil Code 2430-2433 (1983).
Colorado Durable Power of Attorney. Colo. Rev. Stat. § 15-14-501 as amended 1983 by L. 83, p. 661 § 1.

Eichner v. Dillon, 426 N.Y.S. 2d 517, App. Div. (1980).
In re Dinnerstein, 380 N.E. 2d 134, Mass. App. (1978).
In re Quinlan, 70 N.J. 10, 355A, 2d 647 (1976).
In re Storar, 438 N.Y.S. 2d 266, 1981 (consolidated with Eichner v. Dillon).
Klerman, G. L. (1978). Affective disorders. In A. M. Nicholi, Jr. (Ed.), *The Harvard guide to modern psychiatry* (pp. 253-279). Cambridge, MA: The Belknap Press of Harvard University Press.
Kolata, G. (1982). Alzheimer's research poses dilemma. *Science, 215,* 47-48.
Lange, D. J. (1980). Geriatric, psychiatric, and legal aspects of the mental state of the aged. *Legal Medicine Quarterly, 4,* 161-174.
Lessard v. Schmidt, 349 F Supp 1078 (ED Wis 1972).
Makarushka, J. L., & McDonald, R. D. (1979). Informed consent, research, and geriatric patients: The responsibility of institutional review committees. *The Gerontologist, 19,* 61-66.
Meisel, A. (1979). The "exceptions" to the informed consent doctrine: Striking a balance between values in medical decision making. *Wisconsin Law, 47,* 413-488.
Meisel, A., Roth, L. H., & Lidz, C. W. (1977). Toward a model of the legal doctrine of informed consent. *Am J Psychiatry, 134,* 285-289.
Melnick, V. L., Dubler, N. N., Weisbard, A., & Butler, R. N. (1984). Clinical research in Senile Dementia of the Alzheimer Type: Suggested guidelines addressing the ethical and legal issues. *Journal of the American Geriatrics Society, 32*(7), 531-536.
Nolan, B. S. (1984, October). Functional evaluation of the elderly in guardianship proceedings. *Law, Medicine & Health Care,* 210-218.
Pennsylvania Durable Power of Attorney. Pa. Cons. Stat. Ann. §§ 5601-5607 (1982).
Perr, I. N. (1978a). The many faces of competence. In W. E. Barton & C. J. Sandborn (Eds.), *Law and the mental health professions* (pp. 211-234). New York: International Universities Press.
Perr, I. N. (1978b). The most beneficial alternative: A counterpart to the least restrictive alternative. *Bull Am Acad of Psychiatry and the Law, 6,* iv-vii.
Perr, I. N. (1981). Wills, testamentary capacity and undue influence. *Bull Am Acad of Psychiatry and the Law, 9,* 15-22.
President's Commission for the Study of Ethical Problems in Medicine and Biomedical and Behavioral Research (1983). *Deciding to forego life-sustaining treatment—A report on the ethical, medical and legal issues in treatment decisions.* Washington, DC: U.S. Government Printing Office.
Ratzan, R. (1980). Being old makes you different: The ethics of research with elderly subjects. *Hastings Center Report, 10,* 32-42.
Roth, L. H. (1977). Competency to consent to or refuse treatment. In L. Grinspoon (Ed.), *Psychiatry 1982: Annual review* (pp. 350-360). Washington, DC: American Psychiatric Association.
Roth, L. H., Meisel, A., & Lidz, C. W. (1977). Test of competency to consent to treatment. *Am J Psychiatry, 134,* 279-289.

Sadoff, R. L. (1975). *Forensic psychiatry—A practical guide for lawyers and psychiatrists.* Springfield, IL: Thomas.
Salzman, C. (1977). ECT and ethical psychiatry. *Am J Psychiatry, 134,* 1006-1009.
Schloendorff v. Society of New York Hospital, 211 N.Y. 125, 105 N.E. 92 (1914).
Schram, R. B., Kane, J. C., & Roble, D. T. (1978). Law-medicine notes: "No code" orders: Clarification in the aftermath of Saikewicz. *NEJM, 299,* 875-878.
Society for the Right to Die. (1984). *Handbook of living will laws 1981-1984.* New York: The Society for the Right to Die.
Society for the Right to Die. (1986). *Handbook of 1985 living will laws.* NY: Author.
Stanley, B. (1983). Senile dementia and informed consent. *Behavioral Sciences and The Law, 1,* 57-71.
Stone, A. A. (1981). The right to refuse treatment. *Arch Gen Psychiatry, 38,* 358-362. 1980.
Strain, L. A., & Chappell, N. L. (1982). Problems and strategies: Ethical concerns in survey research with the elderly. *The Gerontologist, 22,* 526-531.
Superintendent of Belchertown State School v. Saikewicz, 1977 Mass. Adv. Sh. 2461.
Taub, H. A. (1980). Informed consent, memory, and age. *The Gerontologist, 20,* 686-690.
Tibbles, L. (1978). *Medical and legal aspects of competency as affected by old age.* In S. F. Spicker, K. M. Woodward, & D. D. van Tassel (Eds.), *Aging and the elderly: Humanistic perspectives in gerontology* (pp. 127-151). Highland, NJ: Humanities Press.
U.S. Department of Health and Human Services (1981, January 26). Code of federal regulations, Title 45, Part 46: Protection of human subjects. *Federal Register, 46*(16), 8366.
Wanzer, S. H., Adelstein, S. J., Cranford, R. E., Federman, D. D., Hook, E. D., Moertel, C. G., Safar, P., Stone, A., Taussio, H. B., & van Eys, J. (1984). The physician's responsibility toward hopelessly ill patients. *NEJM, 310*(15), 955-959.

12

Financial Issues Affecting Geriatric Psychiatric Care

Gary L. Gottlieb

The evaluation and treatment of the psychiatric disturbances suffered by older adults are important and interesting. However, barriers to care appear to be pervasive. While stigma, lack of sophistication, and diminishing access to care affect all age groups, numerous issues regarding economic resources and reimbursement are unique to the geriatric population. Providers may be reluctant to provide services for geriatric patients because of frustrations with the complexities of the Medicare system and its associated bureaucracy. Additionally, providers of mental health care are important resources for families in regard to financial issues concerning the care of loved ones.

This chapter provides a detailed description of the financial issues that influence the delivery of mental health services to older adults: prevalence of mental disorders and their importance among the elderly are contrasted with actual public and private expenditures for their treatment and the skewed distribution of financial resources among older Americans. Additionally, the unique characteristics of the geriatric population and the various locations in which they receive care are presented. A detailed presentation of the Medicare system and its resources and expenditures for mental health services follows. Mental health care providers may find especially helpful subsequent sections, which detail Medicare hospital and physician reimbursement benefits for general health services, mental health services, and long-term care. This chapter also presents a description of non-Medicare resources that support the delivery of mental health services for the elderly. An overview of private health insurance policies, Medicaid, and benefits provided in HMOs is included.

This chapter should serve as a helpful tool in day-to-day practice. An understanding of the subtleties of this system can reduce intimidation of providers and encourage the care of this most needy population.

I. General Issues Regarding Prevalence of Mental Disorder in Older Adults, Service Availability, and Utilization

A. As noted in previous chapters, individuals over age 65 account for 11.9% of the American population and consume more than 30% of U.S. health care services (Fowles, 1986). Prevalence estimates indicate that close to 18% of older adults may be suffering significant mental health problems (Myers, Weissman, et al., 1984). A substantial proportion of these disorders are severe or urgent in nature and impose important limitations on overall quality of life: older adults account for nearly a fifth of all suicides, with rates for older males nearly double those of their younger counterparts (Frederick, 1978). Additionally, irreversible cognitive impairment, clearly of highest prevalence in this age group, is considered the single most important factor in the general population's concerns about aging (Secretary's Task Force on Alzheimer's Disease, 1984). However, discriminatory ceilings on third-party mental health reimbursement have skewed utilization of mental health services by older adults.
   1. Individuals over age 65 receive only 7% of all inpatient psychiatric services, 6% of community mental health services, and 9% of all private psychiatric services (Mumford & Siblinger, 1985).
   2. Older adults residing in the community who are suffering psychiatric disorders are significantly less likely to be treated by mental health specialists than are younger people (Shapiro et al., 1984).
   3. Diagnoses of mental disorders account for less than 3% of all inpatient hospital discharges among geriatric patients (Waldo & Lazenby, 1984), and payments for services for these disorders represent about 2.4% of annual Medicare reimbursements. Inpatient care accounted for 83% of total Medicare disbursements for mental health care (Morrison, Janssen, & Motter, 1984).
B. As described by Stein (Chapter 1, this volume), financial resources are unevenly distributed among older adults. This factor affects

utilization and affordability of health care services in this population (Fowles, 1986).
1. More than 20% of older Americans are classified as poor or near poor (a range of income and assets from below the poverty level to 125% of that level). Additionally, almost half of elderly persons who live alone or with nonrelatives are at or near the poverty level.
2. In contrast, median net worth among older adults is well above the U.S. average, and close to 13% of older households have assets that exceed liabilities by more than $250,000.
3. The vast majority of older adults are supported by fixed, passive sources of income, such as Social Security.
4. Only 11% of older Americans are in the workforce, and over half of these individuals are part-time workers. Notably, private health care costs and insurance premiums for the unemployed (retired) and part-time populations are generally borne out of pocket.

C. The elderly usually do not employ traditional mental health resources for diagnostic or treatment services but have substantial need for these services.
1. Medication. Older adults receive as many as 50% of all minor tranquilizers and barbiturates prescribed. Studies have indicated that close to half of all psychotropic use in older adults may be inappropriate or poorly monitored (Gryfe & Gryfe, 1984). However, the NIMH Epidemiological Catchment Area study's (ECA) data indicate that only 1.7% to 8% of all elderly are ever evaluated by a specialist in mental health care (Shapiro et al., 1984).
2. Nursing homes. While only 4.8% of individuals over 65 reside in nursing homes, nearly 23% of people over 85 are institutionalized in these facilities (Waldo & Lazenby, 1984). In 1977 (the last survey from which data are available), 58% of nursing home residents were suffering from disability related to dementia. Additionally, more than 60% of geriatric nursing home residents were diagnosed as having some mental disorder. High prevalance of depression, agitation, abrasiveness, and wandering were reported in addition to disorders characterized as "senility." Patient contact with staff trained to provide psychiatric care and psychiatric consultation in nursing homes is decribed as very limited (Goldman, Feder, & Scanlon, 1986). Therefore, in this age group, an identified high-risk population with extraordinary need for psychiatric services is virtually unserved.

II. Funding Personal Health and Mental Health Care: Medicare

A. Hospital care for the aged is supported by governmental and private sources. Medicare reimbursement accounts for approximately 75% of these costs, with Medicaid, the Veterans Administration, and other government sources each contributing about 5%. Private health insurance benefits cover 8% of hospital care costs, while out-of-pocket payments (deductibles, co-insurance, and uncovered services) are required for the remaining 2-3%. In contrast, nursing home care is largely financed by patients and their families (approximately 50%). Forty-two percent of that bill is borne by Medicaid, with limited Medicare benefits contributing only 2%. Finally, physician services for older adults are financed by Medicare (58%), out-of-pocket payments (25%), private insurance (14%), and Medicaid (3%) (Waldo & Lazenby, 1984).
B. Initiated on July 1, 1966, Title XVIII of the Social Security Act was a response to data provided by the Senate Select Committee on Aging and years of debate regarding national health insurance (Cutler & Fine, 1985; U.S. Senate, 1979; U.S. House of Representatives, 1983; *Medicare and Medicaid Data Book*, 1982; Myers, 1981; GLS Associates, 1986).
   1. Medicare originally covered medical care benefits for individuals over age 65 who were receiving Social Security. The program was expanded in 1972 to include younger disabled individuals and elderly adults who do not meet criteria for Social Security but who are willing to pay a monthly premium for coverage. In 1973, the program was further extended to provide medical coverage for individuals suffering from chronic renal disease. Of the more than 30 million Americans now covered by Medicare, approximately 90% are elderly (about 10% are younger, chronically disabled, or chronic renal patients) (Levit, Lazenby, Waldo, & Davidoff, 1985).
   2. In 1984, Medicare expenditures totaled $65 billion, representing 47% of all public health expenditures and 18% of total expenditures for personal health care. Twenty-one million, or close to 70% of those covered, received benefits, which averaged $3,000 per recipient.
   3. In 1981 (the last year a full data set was analyzed), payments for psychiatric services were 2.4% of total Medicare reimbursements. In contrast, private insurers estimate that 7-18% of their outlays are for mental health care of nonelderly (Morrison, Janssen, & Motter, 1984).

C. Since its introduction, Medicare has provided two independent benefit packages, each funded by its own trust fund.
   1. Institutional benefits. The hospital insurance program (HI), described in most handbooks and policy descriptions as *Part A*, covers inpatient hospital services, home health services, posthospital skilled nursing services (SNF), and hospice care. This institutional insurance policy provides basic coverage for all illnesses. Benefits for psychiatric services are considerably less extensive than those covering nonpsychiatric care.
      a. *Part A* regulations provide coverage for "spells" of an illness. A spell is an inpatient episode that begins with inpatient admission and ends with the close of the first period of 60 consecutive days after discharge. A patient may be discharged and readmitted on several occasions during a spell and still be suffering the same episode of illness, as long as 60 days have not elapsed between discharge and admission.
      b. For nonpsychiatric illnesses, there is no limit on the number of episodes or "total lifetime" inpatient days covered. However, the maximum number of covered days during a single spell is 150 days.
      c. The first 60 days of coverage for each episode are fully paid, subject only to an initial deductible (equal to the estimated average cost of one day of hospitalization—$520 in 1988). The deductible must be met only once during each spell, regardless of the number of readmissions. The next 30 inpatient days are subject to a daily co-insurance payment ($123 per day in 1986), and the last 60 days require an even larger co-insurance contribution (1986—$246).
      d. The last 60 days (days 91–150) of coverage for a given episode are designated as "lifetime reserve" days. This coverage may be used electively during any episode but may be used only once. Therefore, if a patient is hospitalized for 100 days, he or she would have 50 reserve days of remaining coverage for subsequent spells lasting more than 90 days. Patients may elect to save these days for a later date (i.e., for a future prolonged hospitalization) and use other sources (in most cases, self-payment) for payment of any part of days 91–150. Medicare regulations require that a hospital or skilled nursing facility notify a patient of this right at least 5 days prior to the end of coverage and document this notification in the patient's chart.
         (1) If a hospital is not informed that an individual has exhausted all available days of coverage, including lifetime

reserve days, Medicare regulations "guarantee" payment of up to 6 full days of hospitalization.
  e. Among nursing home services, only skilled nursing facility (SNF) care is covered by Medicare. Intermediate, supervised, and domiciliary settings are not reimbursable. SNF services covered are similar to inpatient hospital services. Included are room and board in a semiprivate room, general nursing care, medical social services, physical and other types of therapy, drugs furnished by the SNF, and so forth. Physician services are not covered. Physician services in a nursing home are reimbursed by *Part B* as ambulatory services (see below).
     (1) To obtain SNF benefits, an individual must have been hospitalized for at least 3 consecutive days and must be admitted to the SNF within 30 days after discharge from the hospital.
     (2) Limitations on length of stay are identical to those for inpatient hospitalization.
  f. While there is no limit on the total number of hospitalizations or inpatient days covered for medical or surgical diagnoses, *coverage of inpatient psychiatric services is limited to a total of 190 days during an individual's lifetime.*
     (1) If an individual becomes Medicare-eligible during the course of a first episode of psychiatric hospitalization, Medicare (or its intermediary) may elect to cover less than the full 150 benefit days of that spell. This provision is designed to restrict *Part A* psychiatric benefits to the active phase of treatment and to prevent full reimbursement for a person who may have been previously institutionalized for years.

[Various explanations have been offered in regard to the differentiation of reimbursement of inpatient treatment for mental disorders and coverage of nonpsychiatric hospitalization. From the historical perspective of federal funding for care of the mentally ill, Medicare was considered of minor importance in policy development. The aforementioned 1966 enactment of these benefits for older adult Social Security recipients was less valued by advocates of the mentally ill than the more sweeping Community Mental Health Centers Act of 1963. The virtual concurrence of these developments separated the federal government's commitment to provide discretionary programs for the mentally ill from its health care financing policy. The result has been a dichotomy between services and reimbursement. (1) Care for the mentally ill, especially those who were envisioned as populating (and ultimately vacating) institutional settings, was mandated through federally funded programs in special settings, separate from the traditional health care superstructure. (2) Discriminatory limitations were imposed on federally funded insurance for the mentally ill. Inasmuch as virtually all of the Medicare population is elderly, the ageist impact of these regulations is self-evident (Cutler & Fine, 1985).

Additionally, it was erroneously believed that psychiatric services for the elderly were primarily custodial in nature. Psychiatric benefits were therefore inserted as an "afterthought," subsequent to the design of the Medicare system. As will be evident from the following description, the very complicated formula established to fund outpatient psychiatric care for the elderly under Medicare has actually served to discourage the use of such care (Cutler & Fine, 1985).]

2. The supplementary Medical Insurance (SMI) program of Medicare *Part B* is a voluntary individual insurance program. The coverage is subsidized, underwritten, and administered by the federal government, using local private insurance carriers to assist with administration. Each eligible individual elects whether he or she wishes to participate and pay a monthly premium (approximately $15 in 1985) in partial financial support of the program.

   a. Reimbursement for physician services, consultants, and concurrent care is made according to the "reasonable charge rules." Reasonable charge is the lowest of: (1) the actual charge; (2) the provider's customary charge for similar services; (3) the prevailing charge in the locality for similar services; (4) the carrier's usual amount of reimbursement for comparable services to its own policy holders under comparable circumstances. The carrier [or third-party administrator (TPA)] updates its customary and prevailing charge rates annually, and revisions during a fiscal year are not permitted.

   b. All *Part B* benefits are subject to an annual deductible ($75 in 1986). Nonpsychiatric benefits also require 20% co-payment of reasonable charges.

   c. For the most part, billable services require direct patient treatment or evaluation. However, expenses incurred in obtaining treatment information from relatives or close associates of a patient who may be withdrawn or uncommunicative are reimbursable. Additionally, family counseling services are covered only when the primary purpose of such counseling is the treatment of the identified patient's condition. Allowable family services include: (1) evaluation of the patient's interaction with family members; (2) assessment of

family ability to care for the patient; (3) assistance to family members in patient management.
d. Necessary services delivered under the "direct supervision" of a physician by nurses, psychologists, therapists, or aides are reimbursable under *Part B*. "Direct supervision" is defined as immediate availability to provide assistance at the time of service.
e. Reimbursement for outpatient medical care by supplementary medical insurance (SMI) is not limited by amount or number of visits. However, in designing *Part B* psychiatric benefits, mental illness was characterized as "lacking precise diagnostics and established treatment protocols expected to lead to specified outcomes within a defined period of time" (Cutler & Fine, 1985, p. 20). Therefore, outpatient coverage for psychiatric care was limited to "acute care" limitations. Total annual reasonable charges were set at $500, and the law provided that the most a *Part B* provider could be reimbursed by Medicare for psychiatric care in any calendar year was $312.50 or 62.5% of reasonable charges, whichever was lower. The actual 80% federal share, which is the maximum amount paid by Medicare to the psychiatrist, is only $250 per year.
 (1) This payment limitation applies to expenses incurred for any physician's therapeutic and follow-up care related to a primary psychiatric diagnosis provided to an individual who is not a hospital inpatient.
 (2) Initial diagnostic psychiatric visits, psychiatric consultations, and psychological testing are classified as exempt services. Therefore, charges for these procedures are not included in the annual total subject to limitation. (Physicians may bill for more than one diagnostic visit provided the need can be documented.)
 (3) Services rendered by telephone and visits for the sole purpose of obtaining or renewing a prescription (requiring no new examination of patient status) are not covered.
 (4) Concurrent care is considered to exist when services more extensive than consultative services are rendered by more than one physician during a given period of time. The third-party administrator must decide whether the patient's condition warrants the services of more than one attending physician and if the individual services provided by each physician are reasonable and necessary. Reimbursement for concurrent care requires precise de-

tailed documentation of the necessity of each service rendered.
f. Special reimbursement treatment for the care of patients with Alzheimer's disease (Goldman, Cohen, & Davis, 1985; Financing Subcommittee for Alzheimer's Disease, 1984). Alzheimer's disease has been classified by insurance carriers as both a neurologic and a mental disorder. Two ICD-9 diagnostic codes have been accepted traditionally for these patients (331, neurologic disorder; 290.X, mental disorder). Prior to late 1984, regardless of the content or process of procedures rendered, when physicians' services were coded under the psychiatric code (290.X), they were subject to the $250 federal reimbursement limitation under *Part B*.

In late 1984, the Department of Health and Human Services instructed third-party Medicare administrators (TPAs) to end the $500 annual limit on reasonable charges, as well as its inherent 50% required co-payment, for some outpatient psychiatric services for patients with Alzheimer's disease. The nature of the service provided, *not* the diagnostic code, was to determine reimbursement.
   (1) Charges for initial evaluation and diagnostic procedures continue to be treated separately from ongoing therapy. They are not included in the annual limitation, and they require only 20% co-insurance.
   (2) Medical management of symptoms associated with the disorder and "nonpsychotherapeutic" interventions related to patient and family care are not subject to the annual cap and require only 20% co-insurance (regardless of diagnostic code). However, allowable charges for these procedures are usually less than those for traditional psychiatric visits.
   (3) Psychotherapy visits remain subject to the $250 annual reimbursement limitation.
g. Payment procedures: Two procedures are available for the way that Medicare beneficiaries may receive benefits for physician services.
   (1) A physician may agree to *accept assignment* from *Part B* and, thereby, accept approved "reasonable charges" as payment in full. The TPA will directly pay the provider the approved amount, less co-insurance and deductible. Co-insurance and deductible must be collected by the physician from the patient (or supplementary "medigap" insurance—to be discussed below).

(2) A doctor may elect not to accept assignment. In this case, the beneficiary must present an itemized bill from the doctor in order to obtain the *Part B* "reasonable charge" reimbursement. The doctor must collect the fee and any charges in excess of those deemed "reasonable."
(3) Unless a provider signs a specific agreement with the TPA, stating that he or she will universally accept assignment, the decision to bill in this manner may be made on a patient-by-patient, visit-by-visit basis. Additionally, if a provider agrees to universally accept assignment as a member of a group or hospital practice, that agreement does not apply to fees for patients treated in other practice settings. However, if a physician contractually agrees to always accept assignment (not because of membership in a group or corporation, etc.), then he or she must accept assignment in all practice settings (i.e., office, hospital, consultation, etc.).
(4) "Reasonable charges" are determined related to both a doctor's customary charges and the adjusted prevailing fee for similar services in a particular geographic location. A profile of individual physician charges for specific services is established by the TPA to develop the "customary and prevailing charge" screen with which actual bills are compared. When no freeze on physicians' fees exists, there is at least an 18-month lag before increases in charges are recognized in individual physician profiles. During a freeze, no fee changes are recognized.

3. Recently, provision of Medicare services has been affected by changes in regulations and amendments to Social Security laws. In an effort to prevent depletion of the Medicare Hospital Insurance trust fund, the Tax Equity and Fiscal Responsibility Act (TEFRA) of 1982 imposed sweeping changes in reimbursement for inpatient care. Additionally, TEFRA provided guidelines and provisions for containment of physician-related services (English, Sharfstein, Scherl, Astrachan, & Muszynski, 1986; Frazer, Goldman, & Taube, 1986; Taube, Lee, & Forthofer, 1984).

a. Public Law 98-21, incrementally introducing a system of prospective payment for Medicare hospital expenditures based on a diagnosis-related group (DRG) patient classification system, went into effect on October 1, 1983. The Medicare prospective payment system uses DRGs to establish hospital prices by grouping patients who require similar care. Each inpatient is assigned to one of 468 DRGs. These classifications are derived from principal and secondary diagnoses, procedures rendered, and, to a lesser degree, age, sex, complications, and discharge status. This clinical demographic profile is expected to predict the quantity of hospital resources likely to be consumed during an average hospitalization. Hospital reimbursement is determined prospectively and designated as a specified sum, independent of actual costs incurred. Therefore, payment is considered to be an incentive for efficient utilization of resources. If patients consume extraordinary resources or require prolonged inpatient care, they are classified as "outliers" and Medicare will provide additional payments to the hospital at a reduced rate.

b. Fourteen of the 468 categories established by the prospective payment system (PPS) apply to psychiatric and substance use disorders. As a result of concerns about the accuracy of DRG classifications for psychiatric disorders, a temporary exemption from the PPS was granted to psychiatric hospitals and psychiatric units in general hospitals. Inpatient treatment of patients with principal psychiatric diagnoses in general medical/surgical hospital beds is reimbursed via the new mechanism, even though these patients may be suffering multiple medical and psychiatric illnesses.

  (1) Exempted psychiatric units in general hospitals continue to be paid retrospectively by Medicare. However, TEFRA modified and limited these reimbursements. Incentives for exempt hospitals to reduce costs are apparent: incentive payments are made if the actual cost per case is less than an established target rate. If costs exceed the target, the hospital must absorb the loss; if costs are less than the target rate, the hospital may retain 50% of the difference up to 5% of the target amount.

  (2) Studies of DRG classifications for patients with principal psychiatric diagnoses have confirmed their inaccuracy in predicting consumption of resources. While DRGs account for only a limited proportion of the variation in individual lengths of stay among all diagnoses (approximately 16–40%, depending on the study), they are most inaccurate in explaining psychiatric utilization (approximately 6%) (Frank & Lave, 1985; Taube, Lee, & Forthofer, 1984; English et al., 1986).

  (3) A comprehensive analysis of DRG data (English et al., 1986) strongly indicates that little commonality exists among patients with given psychiatric DRGs. Patients

requiring very short stays are often grouped with individuals in need of longer hospitalization. The study suggests that DRGs favor less severely ill patients and settings that provide short-term evaluation and limited treatment, while penalizing psychiatric units that provide care for substantial numbers of patients with complicated medical, psychiatric, and social problems. The very high prevalence of medical disorders among older adults with psychiatric diagnoses confounds these data. Patients with primary medical diagnoses treated in nonpsychiatric and/or psychiatric units by psychiatric personnel are not considered in any of these studies. Treatment of these patients may contribute inequities not addressed in any current studies. Additionally, the appropriateness of current weighting of secondary medical diagnoses for patients with "principal" psychiatric diagnoses has yet to be evaluated in the literature.

(4) Myriad recommendations for applying prospective payment to psychiatric hospitalization reimbursement are being developed. Formulations have been suggested that recognize psychiatric procedures (e.g., detoxification, rehabilitation, socialization, etc.) and severity of illness as variables in the classification of reimbursemnt for disorders in the same way that operating room procedures are reimbursed under surgical DRGs. Additionally, liberalization of "outlier" policies—reflecting the use of resources for very short stays and extended hospitalization—has been suggested (Frazier, Goldman, & Taube, 1986).

(5) Overall, it is clear that prospective and/or capitated payment for psychiatric services is imminent. It is likely that its form will be adapted from current models, but it is to be hoped that it will address the limitation demonstrated by ongoing research.

c. TEFRA also contains a provision that facilitates the use of prepaid health plans (Iglehart, 1985) by elderly Medicare recipients. The provision allows federally qualified HMOs and specifically defined "competitive medical plans" to contract directly with Medicare. Each month, Medicare will pay such organizations a premium equal to 95% of estimated payment of traditional providers to provide a full menu of Medicare-covered services. While the program allows an HMO to earn its normal profit margin, cost savings above a predetermined

rate must be used to provide extra services on behalf of elderly members.
(1) There is no universal HMO mental health policy. Medicare-participating HMOs are required to provide the aforementioned Medicare-covered mental health services. However, HMO models provide incentives for outpatient primary care (Gottlieb, in preparation). Payments for hospitalization and speciality services are systematically discouraged with financial disincentives in order to control costs. Therefore, many HMOs have little or no provision for specialty mental health service providers. They depend on primary care gatekeepers to triage (at some presumed financial cost to the provider) mental health consultations as they deem necessary. Others contract with groups of "low-cost" mental health providers (i.e., social workers and psychologists) to provide evaluation and treatment of their patients. These groups are also provided with disincentives for inpatient treatment and the use of higher-cost specialists (i.e., psychiatrists). The potential implications of these policies on the psychiatric care of older adults include extreme limitation of access to appropriate specialty care.

[The Omnibus Budget Reconciliation Act of 1987 provides for 50% coverage of $900.00 of outpatient psychiatric visits, or a total of $450.00 a year, starting April 1, 1988. Beginning in 1989, this limit is increased to $2,200.00 a year at 50%, or $1,100.00. In addition, some services by psychologists and some partial hospitalization services will be covered. The new guidelines also provide for brief medical visits that are not subject to the annual cap or the 50% co-payment. These services will be reimbursed at the usual rate of 80%, as are other medical services. The exact formula for this has not yet been published.]

III. Funding Personal Health and Mental Health Care: Other (Non-Medicare) Sources

A. Medicaid: Title XIX of the Social Security Act, Medicaid, was enacted in 1965 to pay for medical care for indigent Americans by providing federal matching funds to the states. While Medicaid does not allow distinctions between psychiatric and other diagnoses, the program does allow states to impose restrictions on types of services provided. It is estimated that Medicaid pays for as much as 25% of all mental health care in the United States (English, Kritzler, & Scherl, 1984; *Medicare and Medicaid Data Book*, 1982).

1. In any given year, between 3 and 4 million individuals over age 65 will receive Medicaid benefits. Most of these people are also enrolled in Medicare. Poor older adults represent 15% to 17% of all Medicaid recipients but account for 40% of program payments. In 1980, the average aged recipient received Medicaid services valued at $2,200, compared to $740 for younger eligibles. In 1982, more than 25% of all aged Medicaid recipients received inpatient (nonpsychiatric and psychiatric) hospital services, 70% were treated by a physician, and four out of every five received prescription drugs (Waldo & Lazenby, 1984).
2. In most states, Medicare is considered to be the primary insurance carrier for eligible recipients. Medicaid generally, but not always, covers deductibles and co-payments for Medicare-covered services.
3. When Medicare benefits have been exhausted, Medicaid may provide reimbursement for services. However, covered services vary and are determined by individual states.
    a. Most state Medicaid programs reimburse inpatient psychiatric care for poor older adults after the 190 lifetime days of Medicare coverage have been used. However, the level of reimbursement varies significantly among participating states. The relationship between DRG payments and Medicaid reimbursement for psychiatric care is being developed.
4. Medicaid programs usually reimburse psychiatric physician services as the primary insurer for Medicare recipients who do not elect *Part B* (SMI) coverage. The level of this reimbursement and its restrictions vary considerably among states. Some state Medicaid programs have SMI (*Part B*) buy-in agreements. These states automatically reduce their own risk by paying for Medicare *Part B* on behalf of impoverished elderly. These agreements account for slightly less than one tenth of all SMI premiums (Levit et al., 1985).
    a. Medicaid will cover some portion of deductibles and co-payments for eligible older adults who elect *Part B* Medicare coverage for physician services. Additionally, Medicaid becomes the primary carrier for outpatient psychiatric services after the Medicare "cap" has been attained.
    b. Medicaid reimbursement for inpatient and outpatient physician services is quite variable among states. Fees are generally set at the state level and may be unrelated to charges, "reasonable" costs, or physician profits. In general, reimbursement for psychiatric services is greatly below prevailing fees.

5. State governments have some discretionary power in the development of service programs covered by local Medicaid programs. States vary in the breadth of resources provided and in the kinds of services reimbursed. However, because of the intensity of state and local participation in programs for the indigent mentally ill, numerous programs may be offered that are *not* covered by Medicare. These include day treatment programs, partial hospitalization programs, daycare and respite care for older adults and their families, uncovered home mental health services, and prescription drugs.
6. While Medicare reimbursement of nursing home care is limited and covers only 2% of chronic care expenditures, Medicaid pays about 42% of the bill for skilled and intermediate-level nursing care. Most states require that individuals "spend down" their assets below a certain level in order to become Medicaid-eligible (Levit et al., 1985).
    a. Medicaid traditionally reimburses at a level substantially below nursing home charges. Medicaid recipients often find placement difficult as private pay patients are favorably admitted. Additionally, nursing homes that specialize in the treatment of psychiatric patients are considered "institutions for mental disease" by Medicaid and are ineligible for payments for beneficiaries aged 22–64. Therefore, "younger" older adults with mental disorders who require nursing home placement will be closely scrutinized prior to admission (Goldman, 1986).
7. Medicaid programs have followed federal initiatives and are rapidly pursuing prospective and capitated payment systems for their recipients. Additionally, numerous gatekeeper models are currently in development or start-up phases.

B. Private health insurance is a rapidly growing source of funds for the health care of the aged. Private insurance benefits account for less than one-tenth of all spending for care of the elderly, compared with more than 25% of that for the general population (Waldo & Lazenby, 1984).
   1. The extent of health insurance coverage for older adults varies by the type of service covered. Close to 60% of individuals over age 65 have private insurance that covers hospital expenses, while about 40% are privately insured for coverage of physicians' services. However, because of the level of Medicare enrollment, most private insurance purchased by older adults is in the form of "medigap" coverage.
       a. "Medigap" policies [e.g., Blue Shield 65 Special, AARP (Prudential) supplemental, etc.] provide wraparound coverage of

established Medicare benefits. They require purchase of *Part B* SMI insurance and usually pay Medicare deductible and co-insurance amounts. These policies are always secondary to Medicare and are subject to the same covered services and length-of-stay limits as Medicare. Therefore, they provide marginal enhancement of psychiatric coverage for older adults. Outpatient co-payments are effectively reduced to 37.5% from 50%, but the $500 annual cap is unchanged. Similarly, the lifetime 190-day inpatient limitation is unaffected by these policies (GLS Associates, 1986).
2. A small proportion of employed elderly and older adults who are not Medicare-eligible have private insurance policies as their primary coverage.
   a. While 99% of private health insurance policies have some level of inpatient psychiatric coverage and 94% have some level of outpatient coverage, there are almost always significant limitations in coverage. Only 53% of private policies cover inpatient mental illness expenses in the same way that they cover other illnesses, and only 7% cover outpatient psychiatric services in the same way that outpatient medical care is reimbursed (APA, 1985).
      1. The reduced level of benefits is usually explained by higher co-insurance (e.g., 50%), maximum charges per visit, maximum annual reimbursement (e.g., $1,000–$1,500/year), and limits on the number of covered visits (APA, 1985).
3. Some private insurance companies are entering the long-term care insurance market.
   a. Several organizations, including the AARP, have initiated membership group policies for nursing home care (Goldman, 1986). These policies may cover two to three years of institutionalization and vary in coverage of skilled and nonskilled beds. Additionally, they provide some coverage of home health services. However, most of these programs exclude "functional" mental disorders, while including some dementias.
   b. Life care communities have been operating in several states for more than a decade. These organizations sell contracts to autonomously functioning, unimpaired older adults. They generally provide independent living accommodations, some food service, and various activity programs. For the contract price and a monthly fee, the purchaser is usually entitled to a large menu of health services and intermediate and skilled

nursing care (generally in the community's own facilities and with contracting physicians and hospitals) as required for the duration of his or her life. Psychiatric services for contract holders are generally limited to those provided by *Part B* benefits.

IV. Conclusion—Summary

A. The prevalence of serious mental disorders among the elderly is high, while utilization and availability of specialized psychiatric services is very low.
  1. Income distribution among the elderly is skewed, and the ability of traditional systems to provide all services to this population is questionable.
B. The great majority of older adults use Medicare as their primary insurer for health care services.
  1. Medicare reimbursement for psychiatric services is limited relative to medical and surgical benefits.
     a. Incentives in the current system encourage utilization of inpatient services and severely limit outpatient care.
     b. Virtually all Medicare regulations discriminate in their treatment of mental disorders as compared to nonpsychiatric disorders.
C. Changes in Medicare regulations have led to the implementation of a prospective payment system (PPS) for inpatient services.
  1. Approved psychiatric hospitals and psychiatric units in general hospitals are currently exempt from this system. Psychiatric services provided in hospitals without exempt psychiatric units are subject to the severe limitations of the DRG payment system.
     a. Studies indicate that this prospective payment system is inappropriate for psychiatric care and may be even less appropriate for patients with combined medical and psychiatric disorders.
     b. Numerous recommendations are being developed to modify this system, as some form of PPS is considered inevitable.
  2. Prospective payment for physician services is currently being scrutinized.
D. Medicaid and private insurers provide varied levels of coverage for elderly mentally ill individuals.
  1. They collectively serve primarily as secondary insurers for Medicare recipients.
  2. Medicaid and private pay provide the principal reimbursement for long-term care.

REFERENCES

American Psychiatric Association, Office of Economic Affairs. (1985). A review of the extent and trends in insurance coverage for psychiatric illness in the private sector, based on the annual Bureau of Labor Statistics level of benefit studies. Washington, DC: Author.

Cutler, J., & Fine, T. (1985). Federal health care financing of mental illness: A failure of public policy. In S. S. Sharfstein & A. Beigel (Eds.), *The new economics and psychiatric care* (pp. 17-37). Washington, DC: American Psychiatric Press.

English, J. T., Kritzler, Z. A., & Scherl, D. (1984). Historical trends in the financing of psychiatric services. *Psychiatric Annals, 14*, 321-331.

English, J. T., Sharfstein, S. S., Scherl, D. J., Astrachan, B., & Muszynski, I. L. (1986). Diagnosis-related groups and general hospital psychiatry: The APA study. *Amer J Psychiatry, 143*, 131-139.

Financing Subcommittee for Alzheimer's Disease. (1984). *Task force report.* Washington, DC: Dept. of Health and Human Services.

Fowles, D. G. (1986). A profile of older Americans: 1985. Washington, DC: American Association of Retired Persons.

Frank, R. G., & Lave, J. L. (1985). The psychiatric DRGs: Are they different. *Medical Care, 23*, 1148-1155.

Frazier, S. H., Goldman, H., & Taube, C. A. (1986). Psychiatry, Medicare, and prospective payment (editorial). *Am J Psychiatry, 143*, 198-200.

Frederick, C. J. (1978). Current trends in suicidal behavior in the United States. *Am J Psychotherapy, 32*, 172-200.

GLS Associates, Inc. (1986). *Summary of relevant Medicare regulations.* Report prepared for the University of Pennsylvania, Philadelphia.

Goldman, H. (1986). Financing long-term psychiatric care. *Business and Health, 3* (4), 5-7.

Goldman, H., Cohen, G. D., & Davis, M. (1985). Expanded Medicare outpatient coverage for Alzheimer's disease and related disorders. *Hosp and Comm Psychiatry, 36*, 939-942.

Goldman, H., Feder, J., & Scanlon, W. (1986). Chronic mental patients in nursing homes: Reexamining data from the national nursing home study. *Hosp and Comm Psychiatry, 37*, 269-272.

Gottlieb, G. (in preparation). Survey of mental health programs for older adults in capitated health systems.

Gryfe, C. I., & Gryfe, B. M. (1984). Drug therapy of the aged: The problem of compliance and the roles of physicians and pharmacists. *J Amer Ger Soc, 32*, 301-307.

Iglehart, J. K. (1985). Health policy report: Medicare turns to HMOs. *NEJM, 312*, 132-136.

Levit, K. R., Lazenby, H., Waldo, D. R., & Davidoff, L. M. (1985). National health expenditures, 1984. *Health Care Financing Review, 7*, 1-34.

Medicare and Medicaid Data Book. (1982). Washington, DC: Health Care Financing Administration.

Morrison, L., Janssen, T., & Motter, J. (1984). *Evaluation of the Medicare mental health demonstration*. Silver Spring, MD: Macro Systems.

Mumford, E., & Siblinger, H. J. (1985). Economic discrimination against elderly psychiatric patients under Medicare. *Hosp and Comm Psychiatry, 36*, 587–589.

Myers, J. K., Weissman, M. M., Tischler, G. L., Holzer, C. E., Leaf, P. J., Orvaschel, H., Anthony, J. C., Boyd, J. H., Burke, J. D., Kramer, M., & Stultzman, R. (1984). Six month prevalence of psychiatric disorders in three communities. *Arch Gen Psychiatry, 41*, 959–967.

Myers, R. J. (1981). *Social Security* (2nd ed.). Homewood, IL: Irwin.

Secretary's Task Force on Alzheimer's Disease, U.S. Department of Health and Human Services. (1984). *Alzheimer's disease* [DHHS Publication No. (ADM) 84-1323]. Washington, DC: U.S. Government Printing Office.

Shapiro, S., Skinner, E. A., Kessler, L. G., VonKorff, M., German, P. S., Tischler, G. L., Leaf, P. J., Benham, L., Cottler, L., & Regier, D. A. (1984). Utilization of health and mental health services—Three epidemiologic catchment area sites. *Arch Gen Psychiatry, 41*, 971–978.

Taube, C., Lee, E. S., & Forthofer, R. N. (1984). Diagnosis-related groups for mental disorders, alcoholism and drug abuse: Evaluation and alternatives. *Hosp and Comm Psychiatry, 35*, 452–455.

U.S. House of Representatives, Committee on Ways and Means, Subcommittee on Health. (1983). *Medicare coverage of emergency response systems and direct reimbursement of mental health specialists*. Washington, DC: U.S. Government Printing Office.

U.S. Senate Committee on Finance. (1979). *Background material on health insurance*. Washington, DC: U.S. Government Printing Office.

Waldo, D. R., & Lazenby, H. C. (1984). Demographic characteristics and health care use and expenditures by the aged in the United States: 1977–1984. *Health Care Financing Review, 6*, 1–29.

Index

Index

Abel, E. L., 56-58
Adler, W. H., 37
Age stratification, 4-5
Aging, normal, see Normal aging
Alcoholism, 130-131
Alexopoulos, G., 194-196
Alzheimer's disease
  Medicare and, 238
  and related disorders, 138-145
Ambulatory care, hospital-based psychiatric, 199-200
American Psychiatric Association, 109
Andres, R., 37
Anemias, 81-82
Angina pectoris, 84-85
Antianxiety agents, 183-184
Anticholinergic symptoms, of neuroleptics, 178
Antidepressant medications, 179-187
Antipsychotic medications, 176-179
Anxiety disorders, 128-129
Appelbaum, P. S., 214-215
Arrhythmias, 86
Assessment, psychiatric treatment and, goals of, 103-104
Auditory changes, 27
Availability of services, 231-232

Baker, F. M., 214-215
Barnes, R., 108-109
Barriers to psychotherapy, 149-158
Barsa, J., 199-200
Bartus, R., 173-174
Beels, C., 199-200
Bell, W. G., 214-215
Benign prostatic hyperplasia (BPH), 93
Besdine, R. W., 94

Bhanthumnavin, 36
Bidder, T. G., 185-186
Biological aspects of normal aging, 25-38
Bipolar disorders, 122-123
Birkett, P., 201-204
Black, F. W., 107
Bladder cancers, 74-75
Blood, diseases of, 81-83
Blumenthal, M. D., 173-174
Bone diseases, metabolic, 79-80
Breast cancer, 72
Brief psychodynamic therapy, 159-160
Briggs, F., 200-201
British National Health Service, as system of care, 210-212
Butler, J., 33-34
Butler, R. N., 104-105, 109-110, 149-150, 151-152

Caird, F. I., 32-33
Calkins, E., 95-96
Cameron, I., 1-2
Campbell, L. J., 204-205
Cancer, 69-75
  sexuality and, 55-56
Canfield, C. G., 197-199
Cardiac arrest, 85
Cardiac disease, 83-87
  and sexuality, 52
Cardiovascular changes, 32-33
Cardiovascular problems, with neuroleptics, 178
Care
  ambulatory, hospital-based psychiatric, 199-200
  chronic, settings of, linkages and coordination in, 192-194

251

Care (*continued*)
  informal family, 209–210
  parent, 8–9
  system of, 190–191, 210–212
Carner, E. A., 197–199
Carskadon, M. A., 30–32
Central nervous system changes, 28–30
Cerebral tumors, 73
Challa, H. R., 95–96
Chapman, R., 58–59
Charles, E., 199–200
Chinn, N. M., 197–199
Chronic care settings, linkages and coordination in, 192–194
Chronic obstructive lung disease (COLD), 87–88
Chronic schizophrenia, 127–128
Class differences, 12–13
Coagulation system disorders, 83
Cognitive therapy, 160–164
  aim of, 161
  appraisal of, 163–164
  contraindications for, 163
  indications for, 162–163
  modifications of, 162
  recent outcome studies of, 163
Cohen, C. I., 200–201
Colonic function, 90–92
Colorectal cancer, 70
Comfort, A., 103–104, 105–107
Community activities, 13–14
Community services, psychiatrist's role in linking of, 200–201
Competence, with respect to specific legal issues, 219–227
Conduction defects, 86
Congestive cardiac failure, 87
Connective tissue, diseases of, 95–96
Consent
  to medical treatment, or refusal, 220–225
  for research, 225–227
Conservatorship, 218–219
Cooper, A. J., 58–59
Coordination, linkages and, in chronic care settings, 192–194
Copeland, J., 210–212
Coronary artery disease (CAD), 84–87
Countertransference, 155–156

Crook, T., 107, 173–174
Cross-cultural studies, 11–12
Crown, S., 58–59
Cultural aspects of normal aging, 2–22
Culver, B. H., 33–34

Dagon, E. M., 47, 48
Dall, J. L. C., 32–33
D'Ardenne, P., 58–59
Davis, F. B., 75
Davis, P. J., 75
de Leon, M. J., 107
Dement, W. C., 30–32
Demographics, changing, 4
Department of medicine, interdisciplinary geriatric evaluation/treatment program in, 197–199
Depression, 114–122
  diagnosis and symptomatology of, 115–117
  differential diagnosis of, 118–119
  epidemiology of, 114–115
  mortality in, 121–122
  pathogenesis of, 117–118
  suicide and, 122
  treatment and outcome of, 119–121
Developmental challenges and tasks, of later life, 147–149
Diabetes, 76–77
Diagnosis-related group, 239–241
Diagnostic process, 109
Disease(s)
  of blood, 81–83
  of genitourinary tract, sexuality and, 48–51
  of joints and connective tissue, 95–96
  normal aging and, sexuality in, 41–45
  pulmonary, 87–89
Disorders
  endocrine, nutritional and metabolic, 75–81
  functional psychiatric, 113–134
  gastrointestinal, 89–92
  genitourinary, 92–94
Docherty, J. P., 194–196

Index

Drugs
  memory-enhancement, 185
  and sexual dysfunction, 56-58
  See also Medications
DSM-III-R, 109
Duodenal abnormalities, 90
Durable power of attorney statutes, 222-223

Economic issues, 14-18
Education, 14
Eisdorfer, C., 1-2, 197-199
Electroconvulsive therapy (ECT), 185-186
  general principles regarding, 173-174
  legal issues of, 225
Electrolyte disorders, 80-81
Endocrine changes, 34-36
Endocrine disease, sexuality and, 53-54
Endocrine disorders, 75-81
Endocrine tumors, 73-74
Environmental issues, 18-20
Esophageal cancer, 70
Esophageal motility abnormalities, 89-90
Evaluation, laboratory, 108-109
Evaluation program, interdisciplinary geriatric, in department of medicine, 197-199
Examination
  mental-status, 107
  physical, 107-108
Extrapyramidal symptoms (EPS), of neuroleptics, 177-178

Failure of temperature regulation, 94-95
Family, developmental challenges and tasks regarding, 149
Family care, informal, 209-210
Family relations, 6-7
Family therapy, 166-168
  indications for, 167
  techniques of, 168
Ferris, S. H., 107, 173-174
Filipp, L., 201-204
Financial issues, 230-246
Fink, M., 185-186
Finkel, S. I., 1-2, 194-196

Fluid disorders, 80-81
Fogel, B., 196-197
Folstein, M., 107, 201-204
Folstein, S. E., 107
Foster, J. R., 37
Fox, R. A., 37
Freeman, E., 33-34
Function
  intellectual, 9-10
  sexual, physical illnesses affecting, 46-56
Functional digestive disorders, 89-92
Functional psychiatric disorders, 113-134
Functional psychoses, 123-128
Funding, of personal health and mental health care
  through Medicare, 233-242
  through other sources, 242-246

Gaitz, C. M., 149-150
Ganz, N. M., 65-68
Gastric abnormalities, 90
Gastrointestinal changes, 36
Gastrointestinal disorders, 89-92
Genitourinary disorders, 92-94
Genitourinary tract, diseases of, sexuality and, 48-51
Geriatric organic psychopathology
  approaches to, 138-143
  etiology of, 143-145
German, P. S., 190-191
Gerstenblith, G., 32-33
Giant cell arteritis, 96
Gleckman, R. A., 65-68
Glover, 58-59
Goals, of psychiatric assessment and treatment, 103-104
Goldfarb, A. I., 151-152
Gottlieb, G., 197-199
Gout and pseudogout, 96
Gram-negative septicemia, 67-68
Gram-positive infections, 67
Grau, L., 209-210
Griffith, E. R., 46-56
Group therapy, 164-166
  techniques of, 165-166
Groves, B. M., 83-87
Guardianship, 217-218
Gurland, B., 199-200
Gynecological disorders, 94

Hargreaves, W. A., 190–191
Harris, T. B., 94
Hatch, J. P., 58–59
Hawton, K., 58–59
Health care, see Care
Health insurance, private, 244–246
Health maintenance organizations, 241–242
Health status, 20–22
Heart disease, valvular, 83–84
Hematological malignancies, 73
Herpes simplex encephalitis, 68
Herpes zoster, 66–67
Historical perspective, on normal aging, 1–2
History, medical, 105–107
Hontela, S., 1–2
Hospital, private psychiatric, 194–196
Hospital-based psychiatric ambulatory care and outreach, 199–200
Hospitalization, legal issues of, 219–220
Housing issues, 18–20
Hydrogen ion (pH) disturbances, 81
Hyperparathyroidism, 77–78
Hypertension, 86–87
Hyperthermia, 94–95
Hypoglycemia, 76
Hypokalemia, 80–81
Hyponatremia, 80
Hypothermia, accidental, 94
Hysterectomy, sexuality and, 50–51

Illnesses, physical, affecting sexual function, 46–56
Immunologic changes, 37–38
Individual psychotherapy
  age-specific issues in, 154–157
  goals of, 152–153
  indications for, 153–154
  in institutions, 160
  process of, 157–159
  specialized techniques of, 159–168
Infections, 65–68
Infective endocarditis, 86
Informal family care, 209–210
Inpatient psychiatric centers, linkages between service disciplines in, 204–205

Inpatient unit, medical-psychiatric, 196–197
Institutional benefits, of Medicare, 234–235
Institutions, psychotherapy in, 160
Insurance, private health, 244–246
Intellectual functioning, 9–10
Intelligence, changes in, 29–30
Interdisciplinary geriatric evaluation/treatment program in department of medicine, 197–199
Intrapsychic developmental challenges and tasks, 147–149

Jarvik, L. F., 104–105, 107–108
Jenike, M., 173–174
Johnson, V., 45–46
Joints, diseases of, 95–96

Kafonek, S., 201–204
Kahana, R. J., 151–152
Kaplan, H. S., 46, 56–59
Karasu, T. B., 151–152
Kass, F., 199–200
Keill, S. L., 206–208
Kennedy, B. J., 69–75
Ketoacidosis, 76–77

Laboratory evaluation, 108–109
Lakatta, E. G., 32–33
Larson, E. B., 197–199
Lazarus, L. W., 149–150, 151–152
Learning changes, 28–29
Legal issues, 214–227
  competence with respect to specific, 219–227
  general principles regarding, 214–215
Levine, S. B., 58–59
Lewis, M. I., 104–105, 109–110, 149–150, 151–152
Lidz, C. W., 214–215
Life, quality of, 224–225
Life-review therapy, 159
Lindenfeld, J., 83–87
Linkages
  of community services, psychiatrist's role in, 200–201
  and coordination, in chronic care settings, 192–194

Index

between public and private sectors, 206–208
between service disciplines in inpatient psychiatric centers, 204–205
Lip cancers, 69–70
Lithium, 182–183
Living Will, 221–222
Lucas, M., 201–204
Lung cancer, 71–72

Male sexual dysfunction, 93–94
Malnutrition, 78–79
Mania, 122–123
Mark, V. H., 201–204
Mastectomy, sexuality and, 51–52
Masters, W. H., 45–46
McHugh, P. R., 107
Medicaid, 242–244
Medical aspects, 65–97
Medical Letter, 56–58
Medical-psychiatric inpatient unit, 196–197
Medical treatment, consent or refusal of, 220–225
Medicare, 233–242
  benefit packages of, 234–242
  initiation of, 233
  payment procedures of, 238–239
Medications
  antidepressant, 179–187
  antipsychotic, 176–179
  See also Drugs
Medicine, department of, interdisciplinary geriatric evaluation/treatment program in, 197–199
Meerloo, J. A. M., 151–152
Meisel, A., 214–215
Memory changes, 28–29
Memory-enhancement drugs, 185
Menopause, sexuality and, 49–50
Mental disorder, prevalence of, 231–232
Mental health care, funding of, *see* Funding
Mental health services, organization of, 189–212
Mental-status examination, 107
Metabolic bone diseases, 79–80
Metabolic disorders, 75–81

Miles, L. E., 30–32
Miller, E., 104–105
Miller, K., 214–215
Miller, N., 1–2
Monk, A., 208–209
Monoamine oxidase inhibitors (MAOI), 180–181
Mustille, A., 192–194
Myers, B., 206–208
Myocardial infarction, 85
Myths, 2–4

Nagel, J. F., 37
National Health Service, British, as system of care, 210–212
Natural Death, 221–222
Neoplasms, 73–75
Neuroleptic malignant syndrome, 178–179
Neuroleptics, 176–179
Neutropenia, 82–83
"No Code," 223–224
Nonketotic hyperglycemic hyperosmolar coma, 77
Normal aging, 1–22
  biological aspects of, 25–38
  current social and cultural aspects of, 2–23
  and disease, sexuality in, 41–45
  historical perspective of, 1–2
  normal sexual response cycle with, 45–46
Norris, A. M., 37
Nursing home, psychiatrist and, 201–204
Nutritional disorders, 75–81

Obesity, 79
Oral cancers, 69–70
Organic psychopathology, geriatric, 138–145
Organization of mental health services, 189–212
Osteomalacia, 79–80
Osteoporosis, 79
Ostomy, sexuality and, 56
Outreach, hospital-based psychiatric ambulatory care and, 199–200

Paget's disease, 96
Pancreatic cancer, 71

Papademetriou, T., 95-96
Papadopoulos, C., 56-58
Parent care, 8-9
Perr, I. N., 214-215, 217-219
Personal health care, funding of, *see* Funding
Personality, 10
Peskind, E., 108-109
Peterson, B. A., 69-75
Pfeiffer, E., 45-46, 109-110, 151-152
Pharmacokinetics, 175-176
Physical examination, 107-108
Pneumonia, 87
Political activities, 13-14
Polycyclic antidepressants, 179-180
Polymyalgia rheumatica (PMR), 96
Polysomnography (sleep laboratory) findings, 30-32
Prevalence of mental disorder, 231-232
Private health insurance, 244-246
Private psychiatric hospitals, 194-196
Private sector, public and, need for linkages between, 206-208
Prospective payment system (PPS), 240
Prostate disease, sexuality and, 48-49
Prostatic carcinoma, 72-73
Psychiatric ambulatory care, hospital-based, 199-200
Psychiatric assessment, goals of, 103-104
Psychiatric centers, inpatient, linkages between service disciplines in, 204-205
Psychiatric disorders, functional, 113-134
Psychiatric hospitals, private, 194-196
Psychiatric treatment, *see* Therapeutic *entries*; Treatment *entries*
Psychiatrist
  and nursing home, 201-204
  role of, in linking community services, 200-201
Psychopathology, geriatric organic, 138-145

Psychopharmacologic therapy, 174-185
Psychoses, functional, 123-128
Psychoses of late onset, 123-127
  differential diagnosis of, 125
  epidemiology of, 125
  pathogenesis of, 125-126
  treatment and outcome of, 126-127
Psychotherapy, *see* Therapy; Treatment
Public sector, and private, need for linkages between, 206-208
Pulmonary changes, 33-34
Pulmonary diseases, 87-89
Pulmonary embolism, 88

Quality of life, 224-225

Race differences, 12-13
Raskin, A., 107
Raskind, M., 108-109
Rectal function, 90-92
Refusal of medical treatment, consent or, 220-225
Reifler, E. V., 197-199
Reisberg, B., 107
Relations, family, 6-7
Religion, 14
Reminiscence, 159
Renal changes, 37
Renal disease, sexuality and, 54
Renshaw, D. C., 46-56
Research, consent for, 225-227
Resistance, expressions of, 156-157
Respiratory disease, sexuality and, 53
Resuscitation, 223-224
Rheumatoid arthritis, 95
Rheumatoid disease, sexuality and, 54-55
Rivaro, M. F., 108-109
Rosenthal, J. S., 37
Roth, L. H., 214-215
Rovner, B. W., 201-204
Rowe, J. W., 37

Sabin, T. D., 201-204
Sadoff, R. L., 215, 217-219
Salzman, C., 173-174, 185-186
Schizophrenia, chronic, 127-128

Schmidt, W., 214-215
Schuster, 36
Secondary sexual organs, diseases of, 51-52
Sedative-hypnotics, 184-185
Segraves, R. T., 56-58
Seligman, P. A., 81
Senses, changes in special, 27
Service disciplines in inpatient psychiatric centers, linkages between, 204-205
Services
  availability and utilization of, 231-232
  mental health, organization of, 189-212
  social, 208-209
Sex differences, 12
Sexual dysfunction(s)
  components of, 46
  drugs and, 56-58
  male, 93-94
  management of, 58-59
Sexual function, physical illnesses affecting, 46-56
Sexual organs, secondary, diseases of, 51-52
Sexual response cycle, normal, with normal aging, 45-46
Sexuality, in normal aging and disease, 41-45
Shapiro, S., 190-191
Shock, N. W., 37
Skin neoplasms, 74
Skinner, E. A., 190-191
Sleep, and sleep disorders, 131-134
Sleep apnea, 88-89, 133
Sleep changes, 30-32
Small, G. W., 104-105
Social aspects of normal aging, 2-22
Social norms, 5-6
Social services, 208-209
Somatic therapies, 173-186
Spar, J., 109-110
Spinal cord tumors, 73
Stein, E., 1-2, 206-208
Steinberg, R. M., 208-209
Stereotypes, 2-4
Stimulants, 181-182
Stomach cancer, 70-71
Stoudemire, A., 196-197

Strokes, sexuality and, 52-53
Strub, R. L., 107
Subentorial tumors, 73
Suicide, depression and, 122
Sumi, S. M., 197-199
Supplementary Medical Insurance (SMI), 236-239
Syphilis, 68
System of care, 190-191
  British National Health Service as, 210-212

Taeuber, C. M., 2-22
Targum, S. D., 194-196
Tax Equity and Fiscal Responsibility Act (TEFRA), 239-242
Technical considerations, 104-105
Teeth, acquired loss of, 89
Temperature regulation, failure of, 94-95
Termination, 159
Testamentary capacity, 215-217
Testimonial capacity, 215
Tetanus, 66
Texter, E. C., 36
Therapeutic relationship, establishment of, 151-152
Therapy(ies), 147-168
  barriers to, 149-158
  brief psychodynamic, 159-160
  cognitive, 160-164
  electroconvulsive, *see* Electroconvulsive therapy
  family, 166-168
  group, 164-166
  individual, *see* Individual therapy
  in institutions, 160
  life-review, 159
  psychopharmacologic, 174-185
  somatic, 173-186
  See also Treatment *entries*
Thyroid diseases, 75-76
Tobin, J. D., 37
Tobin, S. S., 208-209
Todeland, R., 208-209
Toner, J., 204-205
Transference, 154-155
Treatment
  medical, consent or refusal of, 220-225
  psychiatric, 103-104, 109-110

Treatment (*continued*)
  psychopharmacologic, 174–185
  See also Therapeutic *entries*
Treatment program, interdisciplinary geriatric, in department of medicine, 197–199
Trieschmann, R. B., 46–56
Tuberculosis, 66
Tumors, cerebral, subentorial and spinal cord, 73

Urinary incontinence, 92
Uterine cancers, 74–75
Utilization of services, 231–232

Vaginismus, 51
Valvular heart disease, 83–84
Van Arsdalen, K. N., 56–58
Vascular disease, sexuality and, 52–53
Veith, R., 108–109
Verwoerdt, A., 45–46, 103–104, 105–107
Visual changes, 27
Vitamin deficiencies, 78–79
Vitug, A. J., 201–204
Vivell, S., 204–205
Volume depletion, 80

Waxman, H. M., 197–199
Wein, A. J., 56–58
Weinberg, J., 149–150, 151–152
Weisfeldt, M. L., 32–33
Weksler, M. E., 37
Wheatley, D., 109–110
Will(s), 215–217
  Living, 221–222
Williams, B. O., 32–33
Wise, T. N., 46–56
Woodruff, D. S., 30–32
Work roles, 5

Yesavage, J. A., 151–152, 214–215